THE WELL ADJUSTED HORSE

"You take your dog to the vet, and expect him to feel better fast. But if your pet's back is hurting or spine needs adjusting, you're out of luck—most states do not allow chiropractors to work on animals, and only a handful of veterinarians know anything about chiropractic, says Dr. Daniel Kamen, expert on treating anything from sedated lions to llamas. He'll tell you why pet owners should adjust their own dogs' backs, and how to do it."   —*Radio & TV Report* (1996)

"Sorry, he won't do giraffes anymore—but if your dog, cat or horse has a back out of whack, Dr. Daniel Kamen is your man."
—*Star* (1987)

"An Illinois chiropractor is using his skills on animals, and he says the technique works as well on dogs, cats, and horses as it does on humans. An added benefit, says Dr. Daniel R. Kamen of Buffalo Grove, is that four-legged patients don't talk back."
—*Insight* (1986)

"Kamen is a chiropractor with a twist. His main occupation is treating people with back or arthritic problems. However, his sideline is treating animals. He has treated a giraffe, a lion, a bear, a monkey, and several cats, horses and dogs... 'Admittedly, there isn't a big calling for lion chiropractors,' said Kamen. 'You just don't find that many lions or bears in the suburbs.'"
—*Countryside ReminderNews* (1984)

"Though he wants to steer clear of legal beagles, Kamen argued, 'We have evidence that chiropractic works on humans. Animals have similar nervous systems and spines, so I believe chiropractic would help them too.'" —*Chicago Sun-Times* (1982)

The
Well Adjusted Horse

Equine Chiropractic Methods You Can Do

by Dr. Daniel R. Kamen, D.C.

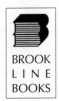

BROOK
L I N E
BOOKS

Reprinted 2001   ISBN 1-57129-063-X

Library of Congress Cataloging-In-Publication Data
Kamen, Daniel R., 1956-
    The well adjusted horse : equine chiropractic methods you can do /
by Dr. Daniel R. Kamen.
        p.   cm.
    Includes bibliographical references and index.
    ISBN 1-57129-063-X (pbk.)
    1. Horses--Wounds and injuries--Chiropractic treatment.
I. Title.
SF951.K3225   1998
636.1'08971--dc21   98-45442
                                                           CIP

DISCLAIMER (to horse owners or anyone else who reads this book): This book
is about managing vertebral subluxations in horses, not treating disease. Do not
use this book in place of veterinary care. All health questions concerning your
horse, including those pertaining to the use of chiropractic care, must initially be
addressed by your veterinarian.

    The author and anyone or anything associated with the writing, production,
or distribution of this book assumes ABSOLUTELY NO liability to or for anyone
(man or beast) who uses the information presented in this book. The reader or
user of the information presented in this book assumes the entire responsibility
and liability for his or her actions.

Illustrated by Jeffrey Kamen. Book design and typography by Erica L. Schultz.

Printed in USA: 10 9 8 7 6 5 4 3 2
reprinted 2001 by P.A. Hutchison Company, Mayfield, PA

Published by BROOKLINE BOOKS
P.O. Box 381047, Cambridge, Massachusetts 02238
Order toll-free: 1-800-666-BOOK • Fax:617-868-1772

Contents

DEDICATIONS

To all the horses in the world ... and other naysayers.

To my wife, Sharon, and my three sons, Jeffrey,
Gary, and Kevin—who not only made this book
possible, but necessary.

* * *

Thanks to my son Jeffrey for his exceptional artistic talent;
to Dick Wetzel and Mike Lacy from the Saddle Barn in
Brown County, Indiana; to the great folks at Green Town-
ship Stable in Cincinnati, Denise Gubser and Jesse Adams;
and to Milton Budoff, Sadi Ranson, Erica Schultz, and Jeff
Mine, the fine people at Brookline Books. Thanks, as always.

Preface

The purpose of this book is to acquaint you, the reader, with chiropractic and its enormous benefit to your equine companion. You will become familiar with healing methods you can perform on your own horse, which will enable you to relieve suffering in the absence of professional equine chiropractic care.

When I tell others I adjust horses, they usually ask, "But isn't that dangerous?" The answer is yes, but only if you're a chiropractor who was caught by the state licensing board. You see, this is the problem and will probably remain the problem for a long time: Not all states in this country allow chiropractors to adjust animals. Therefore, it is sometimes difficult to find a chiropractor willing to risk his or her license to perform this unique service. In one of this country's biggest horse territories, Kentucky, they expressly prohibit a chiropractor from working on horses. In states like Kentucky, horse owners have no choice but to adjust their own horses if they want even limited chiropractic care for their animal.

Equine chiropractic provides dramatic proof of the efficacy of this healing art, evidenced by greatly reduced recovery time following injuries. (This, of course, is also true for human patients.) The number one cause of bodily injury in horses is overtraining. The point is to judge chiropractic for its positive offerings: helping the body restore itself to normal without the use of drugs or surgery. Equine chiropractic care is essential for the trainer who wants that unfair advantage on the track, for the weekend equestrian who wants a smoother ride, and for the dressage competitor who requires more flexibility.

This is the sort of book you have to put down. If you didn't, how else would you adjust your horse?

—Daniel R. Kamen, D.C.
Autumn 1998

Chapter 1

Oh, Wilbur!

Most people my age grew up watching *Mr. Ed*. While many thought there was nothing unusual about a talking horse, I knew the show had to be fantasy. Not that I didn't believe Ed could talk, or that he was smarter than Wilbur—rather, Ed never complained about his back. As an animal chiropractor, I know most horses have bad backs. Why didn't Ed complain about his back? And if he did, who would've helped him?

Animal chiropractic has been around for a long time. As I mentioned in my first book, *The Well Adjusted Dog*, the Palmer School of Chiropractic in Davenport, Iowa, taught a one-month course on equine chiropractic (circa 1921) which was available only to their students. After this one month of training, the students received a "Doctor of Chiropractic Veterinary" certificate. The man at the helm of the equine chiropractic course was the school's namesake, Dr. B.J. Palmer. An entrepreneur par excellence and a carnival barker of sorts, Dr. Palmer enthusiastically embraced animal chiropractic, especially as a way to promote the profession for humans. If it worked for animals, it would work on people, thus satisfying the skeptics who proclaimed that chiropractic adjustments merely provided a placebo effect. This, I think, was the real reason why Dr.

Palmer set up this program. Apparently, the course didn't last long. There is no record of anyone receiving a certificate past 1921.

I presently teach a nationwide seminar on animal chiropractic to veterinarians and chiropractors. Along with a veterinarian, Dr. William Inman of Seattle, I travel around the country to conduct these seminars. We have had an excellent response, often selling out the spaces, and have begun doing three-day seminars devoted to our loyal friend, the horse.

Treating horses was really just an afterthought for me. I learned a little about animal adjusting from friends and teachers while I was in chiropractic college. But when I set up a human practice after graduation, I had planned to work only on people. Still, animal adjusting made so much sense. In fact, it made more sense to my human patients than it did to me during my first year in practice. Since I worked near a racetrack (Arlington Park), I naturally had patients who owned or worked with horses. The question of whether I could and would adjust their horses was often raised. After a while, I finally gave in, took a ride out to the track, and looked at a horse.

When I entered the stall and stared at the horse's size, the first thought that entered my mind is "What am I *doing* here?" Horses are big, imposing, head-butting, kicking machines. If they had the mind to, they could end my career with one solid hoof to the chest. However, most horses wouldn't do that. While horses' temperaments are at times unpredictable, they are generally sweet and gentle creatures. They know when they're sick, and they also know when someone is trying to help them.

The first adjustment I administered to this horse was a complete success, largely due to luck and a little ingenuity. My patient, a six-year-old gelding, had been racing for about three years. "Mister Melvin" performed about average during his racing career, running in the money every three or four heats. His last two races were sub par and he was getting slower. His owner, Bill, who was a patient of mine, told me Mister Melvin seemed to lose his kick in the stretch. The vet gave him a clean bill of health, and there was no apparent lameness. His weight was good, his mood was bright, and his stride was smooth. So what was the problem?

Armed with only human examination protocols, I began to bend and palpate Melvin's neck and feel his spine. Not knowing exactly what I was feeling for, I tried to assess the muscles for areas of stress, or any other evidence of a subluxation. When I couldn't detect any obvious hard spasms, just minor muscle knots, I instinctively lifted the tail to apply a very easy technique called the Logan Basic Technique (see Chapter 13). Administering this move doesn't require a lot of skill. It's a simple matter of locating the sacrotuberous ligament, which is a fibrous band of tissue that can be felt just underneath the base of the tail, and applying a low-force pressure with your thumb. As I grasped the tail and started to lift it up, I noticed it wouldn't move. It was as though the tail was an inanimate object attached to the rump by rivets. I asked Bill whether he had ever observed this. He said yes, that it was due to an injury Melvin had sustained as a foal. He got his tail caught between a metal fence and snapped off the last three coccygeal vertebrae, which are small tailbones.

I was sure Melvin's injury went further than that. Missing a few tail bones would account for the deformed appearance of the tail, but not for a sudden decrease in speed during a race. Or maybe it would! The muscles at the root of the tail connect with the muscles belonging to the sacrum (the bone just below the lumbar spinal vertebrae). Since the sacrum connects with the spine, any stress on the sacrum affects the spine. The fact that the horse was only six years old explains why he performed fairly well during his youth, but now his early tail injury was catching up to him. Since he wasn't properly treated following the injury, the tail was never supple enough to allow the nerves to "breathe." The rest of the lower spine was now faltering due to the tail weakness, thus robbing the hind limbs of valuable nerve flow. It is the hind limbs of a horse, or any quadruped, that provide the powerful thrust necessary for running.

Without explaining to Bill what I intended to accomplish, I started to vigorously knead Melvin's tail with both hands. After three minutes my wrists were so fatigued from pulling and twisting, I had to stop. I resumed, then stopped again to regain my strength. I repeated this treatment pattern for about fifteen minutes. When I was finished, the tail was soft and pliable. Bill, who was watching Melvin's face during the treatment, told me he saw a relieved sigh come over the horse's face like he never saw before, and then Melvin licked his lips. Horses do this when they become relaxed; I often notice this after an adjustment. I checked out a few more areas on Melvin's back and asked Bill to call me the next day with a progress report.

When Bill didn't call for a week, I assumed nothing was the matter. Then he called.

"Hi Doc, Bill here."

"Bill? I thought you were dead. After I worked on Mister Melvin I thought you were going to call me with the good or bad news right away. It is good news, isn't it?"

"Well, yes and no," Bill said.

"What do you mean?" I asked, resonating with a little fear.

"Well," Bill continued, "ever since you pulled Mel's tail, he's been pissing like a racehorse."

"But Bill, he *is* a racehorse."

"You don't get it, Doc. It seems like he's going all the time. Every few minutes another puddle. I called the vet and he seems to think Mel has an infection."

"Does he feel hot?" I asked.

"No, not really. But he seems awfully jittery. Much more than last week."

"I don't know what to tell you, Bill."

"Look, Doc, I'm a little worried. I spent a lot of money keeping Mel here, and now I'm afraid I won't be able to race him."

"Why?" I asked. "Just because he tinkles too much?"

"No," Bill said. "Because he's having a hard time sitting still. Real jumpy."

"Bill, this is not panic time. See what happens over the next week or two. Sometimes the body clears out after the adjustment and reacts in strange ways."

"OK, Doc. I'll be talking to you."

When I hung up the phone, a million things ran through my mind. What if I had actually hurt Melvin? Why did I even agree to look at this horse? I was new in practice and I needed patients. But I wasn't that desperate.

I tried to forget about the whole thing. Impossible. Bill didn't call, and I thought no news was good news. Then I got the surprise of my life.

Reading the Tuesday morning *Chicago Tribune*, I flipped to the sports page and looked at the previous day's Arlington Park racing charts. And there it was. Third race of the day, *Mistermelvin*, spelled with both names blended together, was on top of the chart. He won at 20–1 odds! I was so excited I dropped the paper and immediately called Bill.

"Hello?"

"Bill? I just saw in the paper that Melvin won. At a price!"

"Oh, yeah, Doc. Didn't my office manager call you?"

"What office manager? You don't have an office manager." Bill ran a part-time delivery service (mainly for a local pharmacy) when he wasn't fussing over his horse. The closest he had to an office manager was when his ten-year-old daughter accidentally answered the phone.

"Yeah, well, he did it," Bill said. "Mel won."

"I know. I just read it. Why didn't you tell me he was running?"

"Well, thanks for everything, Doc. Got to go."

With that, Bill hung up.

I'll tell you why he didn't tell me his horse won: because no one likes to share the spoils of a winning horse. Bill was afraid I was going to ask for a piece of the purse. Which I wasn't. I didn't even charge him for an adjustment at the time of the barn call. However, I later sent him a bill, which he never paid. But I learned a great deal that day. I learned that chiropractic works—and not just for people! I also learned to collect my fees in advance whenever I adjust a racehorse.

I once read a very wise axiom. "A man will never commit suicide when he has a sound racehorse in the barn." How true. And I feel that chiropractic is somewhat responsible for saving many a horse owner's life, because chiropractic helps horses perform at their best. Once the secrets of equine chiropractic are revealed, there's no telling how many Secretariats will be discovered!

There was a second incident which strengthened my sense of the power of chiropractic for horses. That was the story of Old Ollie and Little Tom Tom.

I got to know Ollie when I did some work for his boss, Ben Showalter. Ben was a quiet, moderately successful horse owner/trainer who took care of Ollie. Ben gave him a place to stay (a trailer on the outskirts of town) and bought all his groceries. I think he even paid Ollie—but you'd never know it. Ollie never complained. He just liked to talk to people, horses, or anyone else who would listen. And one of the topics Ollie liked to talk about was how he was finally going to win a big race, invest his winnings, and retire. But he had a problem. He didn't own any decent horses. The best of the two nags he had in his barn were probably no more than $2500.00 claimers. Even if one of his horses did win, he would get a little over a thousand bucks. Though Ollie might have been able to retire on that!

One day, during the summer of '83, I was betting at Arlington Park. I was sitting in the stands looking at the racing form and trying to figure out which race wasn't fixed. I'm not sure why horse players rack their brains figuring out who's going to win when many races are fixed. You can't handicap larceny. Anyway, I saw this horse, Little Tom Tom, who was running in the fifth race. His odds were 30-1. He had not raced in over three months and was scratched lame twice the year before. Rule number one in horse racing is never bet on a horse who was scratched due to lameness, the ultimate unknown. But I placed two dollars on this horse and sat down to watch my investment. Tom performed as expected. Dead last. But I was paying close attention to him while he was running. I noticed his right hind leg extended backward just a little less than the left. I also watched him walk during his cooldown after the race. Same thing. Only when he walked, his head and hip would bob up slightly after each step. Something wasn't right, and I wanted to find out.

After the seventh race I left the grandstands. I stopped in the commissary to get some coffee and saw Ollie sitting at an unbussed table drinking a beer.

"You know, Ollie," I said, "I saw a horse run a little while ago that may be just right for you."

"Yeah?" he said uninspired.

"Yeah. Little Tom Tom," I said.

"Who?"

"Little Tom Tom. He just ran in the fifth race."

"Little Tom Tom," Ollie said, shaking his head. "He's the only horse you can bet two bucks on and end up losing three."

"Yes, I know. But he has something wrong with him. In fact, I don't understand why they raced him."

"I don't know. Smithers trains him."

"Do you think I can take a look at him? I mean, maybe there's something I can do."

"Like what?" Ollie said. "Crack his back?"

"Well, maybe," I said rather shyly.

Ollie finished his last swig of beer, then slowly got up from the torn-upholstered chair. "Come with me, Doc."

We walked past three long stables, dodging the hot walkers as they paraded their horses through the intertwining gravel-dirt roads surrounding the paddock.

"Here it is," Ollie said.

I followed him past a few stalls and we walked into a decrepit and cluttered little stall office. Smithers, a plain-looking balding man in his fifties, was sitting on an old milk crate smoking a cigarette and talking on a crusty yellow phone.

"Just a second," said Smithers.

I looked around the nasty surroundings, which were much grungier than I was accustomed to. Even if you think the track makes money, there's no sign of it in the stables.

Smithers finally got off the phone. "What is it, Ollie?"

"Doc here is a chiropractor, and he wants to take a look at Tom's back."

"What fer?" Smithers said as he sort of chuckled.

"Well," I said, trying to speak the language, "I noticed Tom had a hitch in his giddy-up."

"You mean Tom has a bad sacroiliac?" Smithers said, to my amazement.

"Could be," I said.

"Tom's leaving us tomorrow. They sold him for $500.00 to Luke Stables in Huntley. But I don't see anything wrong with you taking a peek at him. It won't do him any good though. Doc Russell was just here last week and gave him a clean bill."

I followed Smithers and Ollie to Tom's stable. He wasn't little, and I'm not sure why they named him that. Smithers walked Tom out of the stall. I crept up to Tom and touched his left withers. He still felt warm from the race.

"May I see him walk a few strides?" I asked.

Without answering, Smithers led Tom outside and down a well-worn walkway. I saw the gimp again, but this time up close. "You see? I said with a high-pitched excitement in my voice. He's favoring his right hip."

"Yeah," said Smithers. "I noticed he does that. But so do a lot of other horses."

I pulled Ollie aside and whispered to him. "There's a chance I can help this horse become a winner. Tell you what, Ollie. I'll rent him for two weeks."

"What do you mean, rent him?" Ollie asked in disbelief.

"Rent him, like a car. This would just be between me and the new owner. I'll be responsible for his health care, meals, boarding and upkeep. This may sound strange, but I'd like to see if we can race him again."

"Race him? We just had the Doc look at him—he's in pretty good health, but he told me his racing days were over. We entered him today just to make sure. After today's performance, I'll be glad if he makes a good trail pony."

"Well, then, you have nothing to lose. I'd like to rent him, or take care of him at my expense for a couple of weeks, maybe three. I think his right hip is bothering him and I might be able to fix it."

"All right," Smithers finally said. "But I can't train him myself. I made plans to work a couple of new recruits. Looks like he's Ollie's."

Knowing that Ollie really wasn't a trainer didn't bother me. He knew horses, and he could train with the best of them if he could stay sober. My job as Tom's chiropractor was to see that his joints moved as they should. This right sacroiliac problem had me a little worried. All the time I was analyzing his gait, I was just guessing. Maybe he had something I couldn't help.

"Now what do you want me to do with him?" Ollie asked as he pulled Tom out of the stall.

"Walk him over here," I said, pointing to a wider area in the barn.

Ollie stopped Tom right next to me. I positioned a new bale of hay next to Tom's right hip. Standing on the hay made me over two feet taller. I set the pointy edge of my palm (the heel of the pinky side of my hand) on the top part of Tom's hip.

"I'm ready!" I told Ollie.

"What do you need me to do?"

"Lift up his rear right leg and pull it back," I politely instructed him.

Ollie did what I asked. As he stretched the back leg backwards as far as it would go, I pushed as mightily and as fast as I could. *Clunk!* Tom's sacroiliac made a huge sound as the joint released.

"What the hell was that?" Ollie trembled.

"Just Tom's sacroiliac," I said. "Nothing to worry about."

I jumped off the hay and asked Ollie to walk Tom down the path outside the barn.

"Looks better already," Ollie said with a surprised look on his face.

"Of course he's better. He was stuck!" I gloated while Ollie and I watched Tom walk without the "hitch in his giddy-up."

"How long will that last?" Ollie asked.

"Don't know. But see to it that he gets some rest tonight and doesn't leave his stall. I don't want anything to happen to him. I'll be around in three days. Make sure he gets entered in a race in the next couple of weeks."

We couldn't enter Tom in a big-money race. His previous races were too slow to qualify for any real purses. But a win is a win, and is often a bridge to the more lucrative races. Still, this was all pillow talk, more my pipe dream than Ollie's because it was I who had something to prove.

The following three days were rather uneventful. I was trying to stay busy in my people practice while Ollie had other things to do as well. Tom was my current hobby—my chance at glory. If I could get Tom to perform, I was made at the track. I envisioned headlines in the local paper: "LOCAL CHIROPRACTOR TURNS LOSING HORSES INTO WINNERS!" I pictured myself sitting in the clubhouse hobnobbing with the CEO's who owned the horses, and getting invited to the back room parties at the Hilton next door—playing poker with the big shots. And to think, all of this depended on Tom's sacroiliac.

I drove to the track a few days later and parked my car just past Gate 9. I entered the barn and looked for my patient. There were a couple of grooms around who could help me with the adjustment. "Think it would be all right if I get Joe to help me?" I asked Smithers.

"Go ask him—doesn't bother me."

I watched Tom walk, and saw a marked improvement in his gait, but he was still a little gimpy. I adjusted him, ate lunch at the commissary, and left.

Joe then took over the training duties for a few days, as neither Ollie nor I could be there, and reported his progress to me. "You ought to come down here, Doc. Tom's a new man! Bullet works today," Joe said with a bit of overdone enthusiasm.

"Does he look like a winner?" I asked.

"Well, he's two seconds faster than last week. That's six lengths."

"No kidding. Did you find out about the race?"

"Yeah," said Joe as I heard him fumbling through the schedule. "Next Thursday—second race."

"Next Thursday, second race it is!" I said with childlike excitement. "That gives us six days to get him ready."

I made sure Thursday was clear, and made it my business to come down to the track every afternoon to look after Tom. Each day was more encouraging than the one before. Tom was looking good and running fast.

Thursday came in a hurry. The race was scheduled to go off at 1:45 P.M. I got to the track at 10 A.M. It was Thursday, which meant the handle wasn't going to be too brisk. The die-hards were there, but the family atmosphere was saved for Sunday.

I drove to Gate 9 to check on my patient. Tom looked good and felt good. Joe cleaned him up, rubbed him down, and there was no sign of a gimp. I, too, was feeling good—joking around with the boys and talking to Tom.

"Are you a fast horse?" I asked Tom.

Joe didn't miss a beat. Borrowing a line from *The Three Stooges*, Joe hid behind Tom and gave his best ventriloquy. "I beat Filly-Mignon in the Porterhouse Stakes!"

"That's good enough for me, Tom. Let's boogie!"

I felt confident. There wasn't much competition in the race. A half dozen bug boys were riding most of the nags. Our jockey was Jorge Rodriguez. He couldn't have been more than 22 years old, but he was a reliable veteran. He had been riding horses since he was two, and racing them since nine, in his hometown—just south of the border. He didn't stand more than 5'1" and weighed less than a hundred pounds. But Jorge was as solid as any man: well-muscled, strong and determined.

The first race ended at 1:22 P.M. with a 30–1 shot coming in. This really perked me up. I figured this was the day for long shots. Ollie and I sat together in the grandstands. The place wasn't half full. We were just one minute from post. Phil Georgeff, the track announcer, finished summing up the field.

"The horses are at the post. They're at the post!" Georgeff said in his spirited nasal cry. "They're entering their stalls."

Tom had the fourth poll (number 4) position. Not a bad spot, but potential early road trouble was always a threat—bumping other horses and stumbling. Georgeff continued summing up the activity.

"Still waiting for Frivolity Foolish, Gray Goose, and Tight Leather Pants. Little Tom Tom seems to be acting up a bit." This didn't rattle me. There's always a horse or two who fidgets at the starting stalls. It just happened to be Tom. Sure enough, Tom finally got pushed into the stall and all the horses were ready for the bell. Georgeff uttered his famous trademark:

"Aaaaand they're off!"

This was it. Tom was running. The race was only six fur-longs—not quite a mile—with a field of nine. I could see a bunch of horses in the distance, but couldn't make out which one was Tom. I'm not the binoculars type. Neither was Ollie.

"Gray Goose is on the lead by a short neck. At his heels is Lonesome Larry, Frivolity Foolish, Sarah My Dear, and Tight Leather Pants."

The race was nearly half over, and where the hell was Tom? Georgeff didn't call his name once. Not once. As the horses made their way around the turn, the crowd rose to their feet and started shouting. Even though the place wasn't packed, the decibels were deafening—like a dozen low-flying jets coming in for landing at the same time. You could just hear bits and pieces of names screeching from the high-adrenaline gamblers. Georgeff's voice was barely audible even though it was being amplified a thousand times by Arlington's powerful P.A. system.

Then I saw number 4. It was Tom! Running three wide around the turn, he was peeling off horses like they were stand-ing still. The neon tote board flashed the horse's numbers as the race continued. With a hundred yards to go to the finish line, the numbers read 3-7-1-4, then quickly changed to 3-7-4-1, then 3-4-1-7. Tom was running neck and neck with Sarah My Dear. With only ten yards to go, you couldn't split 'em. The finish was a little off to my right and I didn't have a clear view of the line.

As the horses rushed to the wire, the lady sitting closest to Ollie screamed, thinking Sarah had won, let out a blood-cur-dling "Yahoo!" I thought Tom had won, but I wasn't sure. The photo sign lit up and we had to wait a few minutes to find out the result.

This was an intense two minutes. Finally, a hush fell over the crowd, the tote board cleared and the winning numbers were displayed, "3" "4." Both numbers flashed at once—DEAD HEAT, another sign flashed. This meant both horses finished first, which cut the winning money in half. Instead of Tom paying 40-1, he paid 20-1. Sarah My Dear was the favorite, and only ended paying 1-1.

Ollie and I met a few days later at the commissary next to Gate 9. I was nursing a cup of coffee and Ollie was finishing his beer.

"I told you Tom would win," I said.

Ollie didn't say much. He sat there fidgeting with some important-looking papers.

"Ollie," I said, "you got any more horses with a bad sacro-iliac I could fix? We can make another winner and go places together."

Ollie finished writing something, stood up from the table and gave me one of those fatherly stares while he put his hand on my shoulder.

"I think you got something there, kid, with that chiropractic stuff. A little too late for me, though."

And so it was. Ollie died less than two months later. But I'll never forget his last gasp of enthusiasm which helped me realize how valuable chiropractic is for horses and the human spirit.

* * *

These stories are true accounts of my early exposure to horse chiropractic. Bumbling as I was, I tried not to lose sight of what I learned in chiropractic school: that chiropractic, along with all the laws of nature and healing, applies to every living soul. The problem I faced in my early professional career was just how to apply this incredible healing art to our four-legged friends. This was easier said than done. At the time, I didn't know many practitioners who practiced chiropractic on animals. The few I knew were scattered around the country, and traveling to them was impractical. Thus, learning how to adjust animals was not only a challenge, but a mission. This mission grew into a passion. And that's what I'd like to share with you in this volume.

For the small price of this book, you will reap the benefits of many years of agony—namely mine! This book only took me a few months to write, but it has taken me years to gather the very best and most effective equine chiropractic methods used by modern-day practitioners of the art.

I can appreciate the temptation for some to jump right to the methods chapters and begin adjusting your horse. But grant me a personal favor and read all of the preceding chapters first. Learn *why* your horse needs chiropractic care; Chapter 2, "The Subluxation," will shed some light on that. The chapters on anatomy and examination will help you focus on specific areas of your horse and will arm you with enough information to carry on a dialogue with your chiropractor or vet. Even if you choose not to adjust your horse yourself, you will realize that you have choices to make when it comes to your horse's health.

Chapter 2

The Subluxation

Chiropractic Definition of a Vertebral Subluxation: The physiological and neurological disturbances caused by two adjacent vertebrae pinching a spinal nerve and its related structures (Fig. 2-1). In other words, a vertebra misaligned on top of another vertebra causes pinching of the spinal nerve in between.

A vertebral subluxation reflects the body's desperate need to respond and adapt to adverse mechanical, chemical, or mental stimuli. The organ victimized by these stimuli—let's say the stomach—will try to send an emergency SOS via the spinal cord to the brain. However, this neurological signal will be blunted by tight spinal muscles gripping and choking the vertebrae that house the spinal nerve belonging to the stomach, thus impairing the "cable" and robbing the stomach of neurological impulses. This, in turn, requires other organs to make up the slack, creating a tremendous strain on the entire system.

Are Subluxations Painful?

This is probably the most important question anyone could ask about chiropractic. But the initial answer to this question is a noncommittal one; sometimes. The subluxation does not always hurt. In fact, they are mostly "silent." When people visit

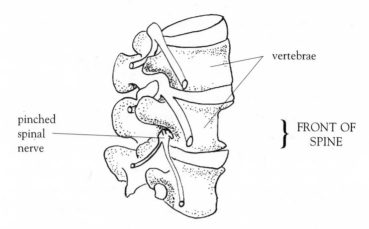

vertebrae

pinched
spinal
nerve

} FRONT OF
SPINE

Fig. 2-1. Spinal nerve pinched between two adjacent vertebrae. (Human
example shown.)

a chiropractor, they don't come in because they think they're
subluxated (although some do), they come in because they're
in pain. By the time someone has pain, the subluxation complex is deeply rooted in the body.

There are seven phases to the vertebral subluxation; misalignment, neuropathy, kinesiopathy, dysfunction, symptoms,
degeneration, and compensation. Note: Sometimes all the phases
can occur within a short period of time (a day or less), and
sometimes the subluxation can fester for weeks or months before the patient comes in with pain or dysfunction.

1. **Misalignment** is the first phase of a subluxation and is
   usually caused by trauma. If a horse bolts from the gate
   and falls, his muscles will splint the traumatized area to
   prevent further injury, and may alter the way he walks.

2. **Neuropathy** is the second phase. This is when the Intervertebral Foramen (IVF) becomes compromised. Because the misalignment closes the IVF, the spinal nerve becomes compressed and less vital.

3. **Kinesiopathy** is the third phase. This is deranged joint motion where the area becomes stiff or fixed. A lot of physiological changes take place here including joint swelling, scarring, adhesion formation, vascular (blood vessel) stress, and muscle atrophy. It is also possible for kinesiopathy to mean excess joint motion (hypermobility). If the initial trauma caused tissue damage (such as a tear), the ligaments may become weak and loose.

4. **Dysfunction** is when the joints and tissues (muscles) don't perform as they should. Limping, head bobbing, and an abnormal gait are signs of dysfunction.

5. **Symptoms** are what bring the patient in the door. *Pain* is the operative word here. Predictably, by the time you see the patient in pain, the subluxation process is already four phases deep and is now part of the body. This is why you have to catch the subluxations in the early stages: *Prevention.*

6. **Degeneration** is one step past pain. Disease and tissue destruction ensues. By this time the patient needs your help whether he wants it or not. It is at this phase that a non-believer in chiropractic becomes an evangelist after the treatment.

7. **Compensations** are often mistaken for subluxations since they share similar characteristics such as muscle

spasms and restricted motion. An example of a compensation is when you subluxate your lower back and then have to twist your upper back while you walk (to lessen the pain). Your upper back is the area that compensates for your lower back pain. The property of a subluxation that's generally missing from a compensation is heat. A true spinal subluxation will feel warm, because heat denotes inflammation, which is one of the signs of a pinched spinal nerve.

Primary Causes of Equine Subluxations

It is just about impossible to pinpoint one primary cause of equine subluxations. But there's one thing for sure: the overwhelming majority of my equine patients suffer from muscle and joint pain, as opposed to visceral disorders caused by toxicity which are more often seen with cats.

In *The Well Adjusted Cat*, I mentioned poisons, such as the preservatives contained in cat food, as a leading cause of feline subluxations. While ingesting poisons can cause subluxations in horses, it certainly isn't epidemic. The majority of vertebral subluxations stem from the horse's body compensating for foot (hoof), ankle (hock), and leg problems and associated lameness. There are also more objective causes of equine subluxations created by man: improper riding styles, ill-fitting saddles, unhealthy stable conditions, overtraining and overfeeding (obesity). Let us first take a brief look at how poisons can cause subluxations before examining the musculoskeletal origins.

How Poisons Cause Subluxations

Poisons or toxins cause subluxations from the inside out—as opposed to the outside in, as with injuries. To understand how poisons or other toxins can cause that "kink" in your spine called the subluxation, I'd like to refer back to a quote by Dr. Daniel David Palmer, the founder of chiropractic. Dr. Palmer wrote about the "one question [that] was always uppermost in my mind in my search for the cause of disease. I desired to know why one person was ailing and why his associate, eating at the same table, working in the same shop, at the same bench, was not." The point is that everyone is born with strengths and weaknesses. Why do some people develop heart disease from eating too much fat, while others can eat five corned beef sandwiches a day for 60 years and be fine? Why do some smokers get cancer and others don't? If there's one lesson I've learned in my 17 years of practice, it's that you can't beat good genes. If you are genetically programmed to get sick at an early age, you will. This is true most of the time. Of course, eating right and exercising can make a difference. And a well-timed open-heart bypass operation can add years to your life. But for the most part, we're doomed. The best you can do is take control of the things you can, and don't worry about the rest.

Now how does this relate to your horse? Horses who are left to graze may accidentally eat certain poisonous plants. Although plant poisoning is not common, it does occur, and sometimes with disastrous or fatal results. Among the more common poisonous plants found in the western United States are *common groundsel*, which can cause permanent liver damage and *yellow star thistle*, which affects the brain. An ornamental plant that is known to cause death by stopping the horse's heart is the *yew*, which is characterized by dark green needles above, a lighter shade of green needles below, and a seed contained in a red, fleshy cup. A horse can die if he consumes as little as 3 or 4 ounces of this plant. Another ornamental plant that is toxic to horses is *oleander*. Ingesting this plant can cause diarrhea, colic, convulsions, irregular heartbeat, and death.

Conscientious owners are aware of poisonous plants in and around their corrals and pastures and take measures to control this vegetation. However, some owners neglect to discourage their horse from eating potentially dangerous house and farmyard shrubs. Additionally, since many people use their horses to ride in the wilderness, their horse may become hungry and eat any available shrub along the way. A couple of toxic plants often seen during packing trips are *rhododendrons* and *azaleas*, which can cause severe colic and diarrhea.

Poisonous plants are not palatable to horses, and they generally avoid them. But horse owners may unwittingly be feeding their animals toxic food if the food product is cubed or pelleted. Food in this form may contain poor quality hay laced with weeds or toxic plants that the horse cannot detect since the toxin is diluted. The bottom line here is that you really have to trust your feed dealer to deliver a quality product.

From the above examples, you can see how the subluxation pattern begins to emerge. If a toxic plant such as common groundsel causes liver damage, then those spinal nerves which control the liver (the mid- to lower back spinal nerves) will become stressed and subluxated. Now the horse has a major organ, the liver, that isn't functioning properly. So what happens now? The rest of the body has to make up the slack. Unless the *cause* of the disease is identified and arrested, ill health will be perpetuated.

As I mentioned earlier, the bulk of my equine patients suffer from lameness due to foot and leg disorders, which in turn cause vertebral subluxations. Appendix A (p. 273) lists some of the more common equine conditions which can cause subluxations. A horse is so large and muscular that just about any physical activity can potentially stress the horse's frame and cause subluxations. But horses are domestic animals and are subject to man's whims, enjoyments, and devices, some of which are detrimental to the animal's health.

Equine Subluxations Caused by Man

For the most part, horse owners take excellent care of their animals. In fact, they are among the most knowledgeable animal handlers in the world. They have to be. It's an enormous responsibility to care for a horse. But in our quest to enjoy them, a few of our implements and habits can slow them down and cause them pain.

1. **Improperly fitting saddles.** This is the number one cause of subluxations in riding horses. A saddle is originally fitted to accommodate the body type of *one* rider. Providing your saddle was bought at a shop where the proprietor knew his or her business, everything should be fine. But when a trail horse is rented out to dozens of different vacationers each year for horseback riding,

the saddle is no longer custom fit and will stress the horse's back in several areas. The padding, shape, and quality of leather used to make the saddle all contribute to its stress factors.

2. **Obesity.** Both of the horse and rider. An obese horse who is forced to be active will suffer from more musculoskeletal disorders, including subluxations, than a trim one. Likewise, a very obese rider can cause severe and chronic back pain in their horse. Some owners mistakenly think they have to overfeed the foals to help them grow. However, this just leads to an obese foal and creates weak legs.

3. **Mounting.** Riders almost always mount their horse from its left side. This drags the left shoulder, thoracic side down, causing muscle weakness there. Incidentally, the other kind of mounting, as in mating, can also cause subluxations of each partner if the mare isn't especially receptive.

4. **Pulling on the leads.** A horse with a right-handed rider will experience more right jaw (TMJ) and right neck pain, because that rider subconsciously pulls harder with their dominant hand. However, yanking on the leads too hard by anyone can stress any upper body joint, especially the neck and jaw. An ill-fitting bit can also cause neck and jaw problems.

5. **Confinement.** Unfortunately, this is a necessary evil. Domestic horses must be kept in stalls for their own protection and security. But ideally, except for resting due to medical reasons, a horse should be free to walk,

run and stretch out. It is impossible to maintain muscle tone and healthy blood flow without regular exercise. *Confinement causes misalignment.*

6. **Transporting your horse.** This is one of reasons why the animal chiropractor must drive all the way to a remote barn to treat his patient. Horses get sore and subluxated in transit. Bumpy rides force their muscles to strain in painful contortions to maintain their balance. This is why I will never bet on a horse who is not stabled at the racetrack. If I notice that a horse (even the favorite) was shipped in for the race that day, I will not bet on him. And most of the time, I'm right!

7. **Racing.** The actual act of horse racing (flats) can cause subluxations, but these are generally due to sloppy track conditions and accidents (bumping into other horses or the rail). Harness racing poses different problems. Horses used for harness (sulky) racing are Standardbreds turned into pacers or trotters; they are fitted with hobbles which are used to purposely alter their gait. Devices such as these will invariably cause leg and back stress over a period of time. The other cause of subluxations in harness horses is running around a small track during the race or training. A mile race over a half-mile oval will compel the horse to make eight turns during the race, as opposed to four turns with a mile oval. The more turns the horse has to make, the more stress he'll put on the inside legs. People who run long distances around small indoor health club tracks often experience back and knee pain, especially if they

have to circle the track sixteen times to finish a mile.

8. **Improper shoeing.** This subject alone can fill volumes. The importance of finding a qualified farrier cannot be overstated. Improper shoeing for any equine event or purpose can cause or worsen any type of equine lameness.

Chapter 3

The Horse's Body:
Bones, Joints, Muscles, & Nerves

Adjusting a horse (Fig. 3-1a) isn't nearly the monumental task you might envision, once you know where to push. When you stand back and observe its massive structure all at once, you'll probably realize how a male Chihuahua feels who's in love with a female Great Dane. But knowledge will set you free. This is not the David vs. Goliath task you think it is. Don't forget, a horse is still composed of parts. Big parts, yes, but parts nonetheless. It is my opinion that in most situations, horses are actually easier to adjust than dogs and cats. The reason for this is threefold:

1. Horses, unlike dogs, generally come in one size, *big*, which makes adjusting techniques predictable (dogs can weigh from less than 3 pounds to over 200 pounds).
2. Horses, unlike cats, usually don't thrash around as much and can't easily run away during the treatment.
3. This may be the best reason: Since horses are so big, you don't feel you can hurt them with the adjusting thrust, thus giving you confidence. I often hear this from the vets and chiropractors who attend my seminars.

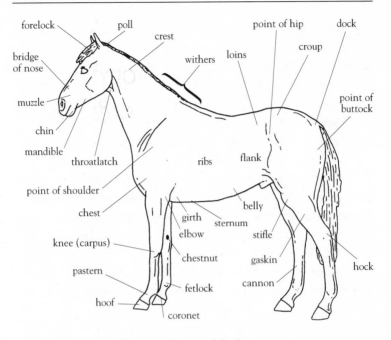

Fig. 3-1a. Points of the horse.

Another reason why I feel horses are easier to adjust than small animals is because their bones are so easy to palpate, even on the bulky draft horse. Later, while reviewing the methods, always keep in mind that speed is the physical component you need to perform the adjustment—not brute force.

Musculoskeletal is a compound word encompassing body parts belonging to the skeleton (bones), muscles, joints, and related soft tissues such as ligaments, tendons and nerves. A *ligament* is a tough fibrous tissue which holds two or more bones together, thus forming a joint. A *tendon* is inelastic fibrous tissue that connects a muscle to a bone. For example, your Achilles tendon (the thickest and strongest tendon on the body) connects with your calf (lower leg) muscles and anchors them into the heel of your foot (Fig. 3-1b). *Nerves* are tissues that detect sensations and motion, energize muscles and organs, and convey impulses between the brain or spinal cord and all the other parts of the body.

While studying the structure of the horse, pay close attention to how the bones relate to each other, namely as joints. Remember, chiropractic is not about setting bones or fractures. Orthopedic surgeons do that. What chiropractic *is* about is restoring normal joint function wherever possible, with your eye on removing vertebral subluxations in particular. A joint not riddled with arthritis or disease still has a chance to return

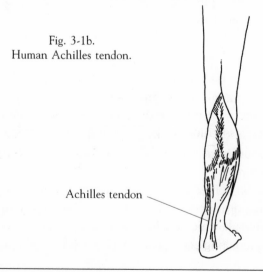

Fig. 3-1b.
Human Achilles tendon.

Achilles tendon

to normal. Also keep in mind that by restoring normal joint function, you are helping to restore normal soft tissue function, mainly nerves, muscles and ligaments. Functionally sound soft tissues are the integral components of good health.

You should read this section with your horse at your side. The diagrams only give you a two-dimensional perspective of your horse, while standing with your horse at your side will give you *bots*.

A horse's skeleton is comprised of a series of short as well as long levers (bones). The long levers provide an extra advantage to the adjuster. The true long bones are found in the legs; humerus, femur, cannon, etc. An example of a pseudo-long lever bone found in the spine would be an upper thoracic (dorsal) vertebra (see Fig. 3-2). Even though the vertebrae are classified as irregular bones, upper thoracic vertebrae contain a spinous process (spine) which is considerably longer than its counterpart found in the lower back (lumbar region). Thus, this upper dorsal bone is easier to grasp, which makes it easier to manipulate. The summit of this bone is about a foot away from the ribs below.

The following pages briefly describe the horse's musculoskeletal system. It is important that you have a working knowledge of the gross structure of the bones along with the strategic adjusting points. This will enable you to integrate both chiropractic technique and muscle therapy, which is an important part of equine chiropractic.

There's nothing worse than a book that tortures you with agonizing details which the reader soon forgets, or the student memorizes just long enough to take the test. It's like watching

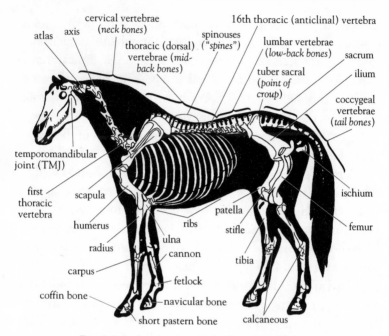

Fig. 3-2. Left side view of the horse's skeleton.

the *Academy Awards* and waiting all night for the winners to be announced. With this in mind, let us review some of the more important aspects of equine anatomy as it relates to adjusting horses. For the true insomniac who insists on turning over every stone (or hoof), I direct you to Sisson and Grossman's *The Anatomy of the Domestic Animals* (W.B. Saunders Co.).

Bones and Joints

The horse has 205 bones, give or take a few. The vertebral column is composed of about 54 bones: 7 cervicals (neck bones), 18 thoracics/dorsals (mid-back bones), 6 lumbars (lower back bones), 5 fused sacral bones, and 15-21 caudal or coccygeal bones (tail). There are 36 ribs, 1 sternum (breast bone), 34 bones in the skull including the auditory (inner ear) ossicles, 40 bones of the thoracic limbs (front legs and appendages) and 40 bones comprising the pelvic limbs (hindquarters and legs). There are some exceptions. The Arabian has 1 fewer lumbar, 1 or 2 fewer thoracics, and a few less tail bones, which would account for their higher tail carriage. Other equines that have 5 lumbars instead of 6 are the donkey, ass, and mule, and the Przewalski, a wild horse that was discovered in the northwest corner of Mongolia by a Russian explorer in 1879. The number of fused sacral bones may also vary among species.

The bones by themselves are of secondary clinical importance as regards the practice of chiropractic. If you were simply a "big bag of bones" with no distinct form or structure, I, as a chiropractor, wouldn't be able to help you. (But my colleague down the street would, providing you had good insurance.) Only when a bone meets (articulates) with another bone to form a joint will chiropractic care be useful.

A joint that bends (flexes or closes) and straightens (extends or opens) with minimal effort, such as the ones formed by the long bones (front and hind limbs), is considered normal even with the presence or expression of pain.

An example of flexion is when you bend your elbow to show someone your muscle (biceps). An example of extension is when you straighten out your elbow to punch that someone in the nose.

The Vertebral Column

The horse's vertebral column, also known as the spinal column, is divided into three areas: neck (cervicals), mid-back (thoracics/dorsals), and lower back (lumbars). The sacrum, which is located directly below the last lumbar, is often considered part of the vertebral column, as are the numerous tail bones (see Fig. 3-2).

The most fundamental structural difference between a human and a horse (or any quadruped) is the attitude of the spinal curves, which affects the distribution of body weight. A human is bipedal and walks erect; therefore, his weight is controlled and supported at the hips. A horse walks on four feet, and more than half of his body weight is supported by the front legs (*thoracic limbs*). This is in part because the front section of the horse has the additional burden of supporting the horizontal head and protecting the vulnerable neck components. Additionally, the horse's spinal column is curved differently from ours. Humans are born with one major spinal curve, a *dorsal arch*. At about age one when walking commences, we develop two secondary spinal curves: one in our neck and the other in the lower back (Fig. 3-3). We maintain the dorsal arch in our mid-back. These secondary curves are also known as *lordotic curves*, and influence our gait during locomotion. A horse has only one secondary curve, which is located in the lower

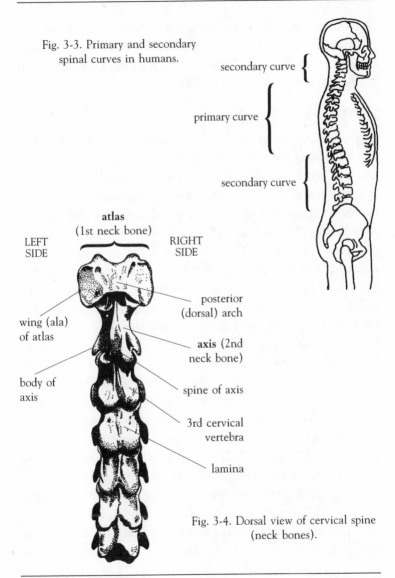

Fig. 3-3. Primary and secondary spinal curves in humans.

secondary curve

primary curve

secondary curve

atlas
(1st neck bone)

LEFT
SIDE

RIGHT
SIDE

posterior
(dorsal) arch

wing (ala)
of atlas

axis (2nd
neck bone)

body of
axis

spine of axis

3rd cervical
vertebra

lamina

Fig. 3-4. Dorsal view of cervical spine
(neck bones).

part of the neck. This accounts for why some human chiro-practors have difficulty adapting human techniques on animals—the angles of a quadruped's body and the direction of the adjusting impulse are different.

Cervical Vertebrae (Neck Bones)

The horse has seven neck bones, called *cervicals*. The only two mammals not possessing seven cervicals are the manatee (sea cow) and the three-toed sloth, who have six.

The first cervical vertebra is called the *atlas*. It is an irregularly shaped, strong ring-like bone which acts as a pedestal that supports the globe (head) and is situated directly below the base of the skull (occiput). The two areas of the atlas that serve as adjusting contact points are the wings (ala) and the posterior arch (see Fig. 3-4). The right and left atlas wings can be seen and easily palpated on each side. By simply walking up to your horse and applying light pressure over the skin on one side beneath the skull, you will expose and feel a clearly demarcated bony outline about the size of your fist (Fig. 3-5). The posterior arch can be felt directly below the poll (base of the skull/occiput).

The joint between the atlas and the occiput is referred to as the "Yes" joint, because it allows for extension (lifting the head up—Fig. 3-6a) and flexion (head bending towards the chest—Fig. 3-6b). However, this head movement is limited in the horse because of occipital projections called *condyles* which penetrate the atlas ring, thus restricting extension. By comparison, a dog has considerable head extension and can literally point his nose directly at the ceiling. A horse has about half to two-thirds this extension range. Later,

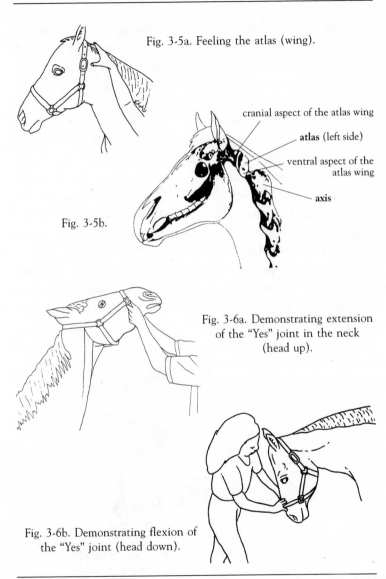

Fig. 3-5a. Feeling the atlas (wing).

cranial aspect of the atlas wing

atlas (left side)

ventral aspect of the atlas wing

axis

Fig. 3-5b.

Fig. 3-6a. Demonstrating extension of the "Yes" joint in the neck (head up).

Fig. 3-6b. Demonstrating flexion of the "Yes" joint (head down).

you will learn to motion out this joint to discern fixations (stuck joints), which are the areas that need to be adjusted.

The vertebra directly below the atlas is the *axis*, or second cervical vertebra (Fig. 3-7). Collectively, the atlas and the axis are known as the upper cervicals; they are markedly distinct from the remaining cervicals. The axis has a frontal emanating projection known as the *dens* or the *odontoid process*. This projection fits into the atlas ring and allows for rotational movement of the head, and is therefore referred to as the "No" joint. The axis also has a large, blade-like spinous process of which the very top ridge can be felt just below the atlas (Fig. 3-8). All the cervical vertebrae, except the atlas, possess a spinous process. However, in a horse, the spinous of the axis is the only one that can be palpated. All the other spinouses are situated too deeply within the cervical musculature to be felt. **Note:** The spinous processes of all the vertebrae are generally referred to simply as the "spines." During the course of

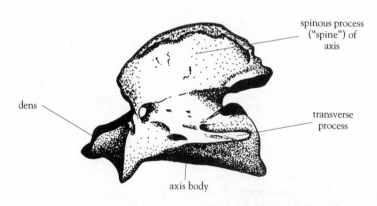

Fig. 3-7. Second cervical vertebra: the axis. (Left view.)

this discussion I will use these two words interchangeably.

All the cervical vertebrae, with the exception of the atlas, have a *body* (see Fig. 3-4). Projections emanating from the sides of the bodies include *transverse processes* and the *lamina-pedicle* junction, which is used as an adjusting contact point for all of the cervicals except the atlas (Fig. 3-9).

Important Anatomical Consideration: Since most equine cervical adjusting is performed with the practitioner stand-

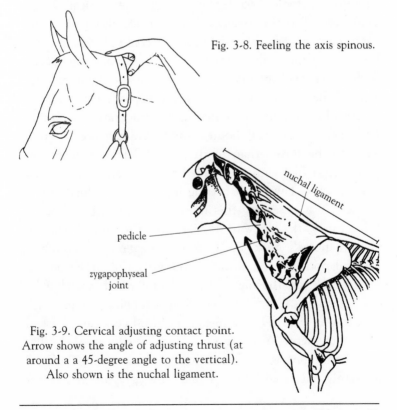

Fig. 3-8. Feeling the axis spinous.

pedicle

zygapophyseal joint

nuchal ligament

Fig. 3-9. Cervical adjusting contact point. Arrow shows the angle of adjusting thrust (at around a a 45-degree angle to the vertical). Also shown is the nuchal ligament.

ing to the side of the horse's neck, you must take into account the angle of the joint *facets*. Facets are flat (with some variations) articulating surfaces found between two vertebrae that allow for joint motion. The adjusting force or thrust is directed along the plane line of the facets—even though the facets themselves cannot be felt (see Fig. 3-9). In the cervical spine, except for the atlas, the facets belonging to the vertebra above meet with the facets of the vertebra below to form a 45-degree angle to the vertical. These joints are called the *zygapophyseal joints*. Knowing this, the practitioner angles his hand and arm accordingly in line with this angle, which allows for a smoother adjustment—going "with the grain of the plane" and not jamming the joint. The angle of the thrust is thus toward the opposite ear.

Another important anatomical consideration is where the cervical vertebral bodies are felt. They are situated closer to the throat than to the mane! I'll never forget an experience I had with a so-called trained practitioner. Back in 1981 when I was still cutting my teeth in animal chiropractic, I was observing this individual adjusting a horse at Arlington Park. He was showing me the "right" way to adjust a horse's neck. As I stood back and observed the master, I noticed his adjusting hand was awfully high on the horse's neck, on the mane. I asked him which vertebra he was adjusting. "C-3," he said while whipping his patient's neck to one side. "Do you mean the third cervical?" I asked with amazement. "Yes," he said, "C-3." I continued, "What part of the bone is your adjusting hand contacting?" "C-3," he sternly reiterated. "But," I said, "the body of that vertebra is nowhere near the mane. It's lower—much lower. It's not even in the same area code as the mane." I didn't say another word. I thought maybe that horse was from Texas. Everything is bigger in Texas, even cervical bodies. But the moral of this story is that when you want to feel the cervical bodies, start at the throat and work your way up. You will feel these projections about a third of the way up from the throat.

It isn't just the angle of the facets that account for the movement of the cervical joints. Ligaments play an important role—possibly the most important role. They are the tissues that unite the bones into joints and provide stability and flexibility to the spine. I will mercifully spare you the intricate details of all the ligaments. For that, you can explore the references at the back of this book. But I would like you to consider two important ligaments; the *ligamentum nuchae* and the *intervertebral discs*.

Nuchal Ligament

As mentioned earlier, the lower part of the horse's neck contains a secondary curve (lordosis). This curve, formed by a series of joints, is really a correction in the spine as it relates to the weight of the head and the pull of the *ligamentum nuchae*. The ligamentum nuchae (a.k.a. nuchal ligament) is a strong elastic apparatus which assists the extensor muscles of the head and neck (raising the head). It attaches to the base of the skull (occiput) and to the top of the withers, as shown in Fig. 3-9. Since the horse's head is really a loaded beam, it needs the support of this ligament to maintain even biomechanics while standing and during locomotion. This ligament acts as a muscular raphe, separating the right and left halves of the cervical muscles, and will often prevent muscle spasms from "bleeding" over to the other side. It is the suspension bridge of the neck.

Intervertebral Discs

The discs or *intervertebral discs* (fibrocartilages) are also classified as ligaments and can be found between the bodies of two adjacent vertebrae and are intimately attached to these structures. They are not found between the atlas and the axis. A disc is a fibrous ligament with a fluid center called the *nucleus pulposus* (Fig. 3-10a). The purpose of the disc is to give shape to the spine, separate the vertebrae, and absorb shock while walking and jumping. The disc is also the site of many types of human back conditions, since it is somewhat prone to injury. A "slipped" or ruptured disc, for example, is when the fluid center (nucleus) bursts out of

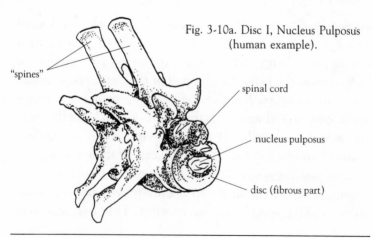

Fig. 3-10a. Disc I, Nucleus Pulposus (human example).

"spines"

spinal cord

nucleus pulposus

disc (fibrous part)

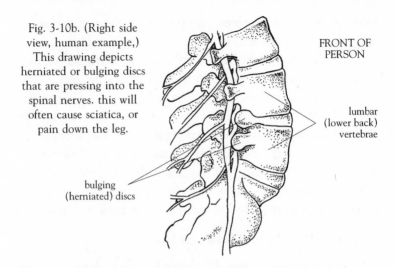

Fig. 3-10b. (Right side view, human example,) This drawing depicts herniated or bulging discs that are pressing into the spinal nerves. this will often cause sciatica, or pain down the leg.

FRONT OF PERSON

lumbar (lower back) vertebrae

bulging (herniated) discs

the surrounding fiber and oozes into a spinal nerve (Fig. 3-10b). The discs are thickest in the cervical spine and coccygeal (tail) region. They are relatively thin in the mid-back (thoracic region). In other words, the discs are thickest in the spinal areas with the greatest movement.

The chiropractic practitioner should use caution when treating an animal with a herniated disc, such as a dog or cat. But slipped discs *do not occur* in horses! In most large animals such as horses, the disc is composed almost entirely of tough, fibrous tissue, with almost no "soft center," which is the part that oozes out of the vertebral boundaries and into a spinal nerve in man and smaller animals. However, the horse's cervical discs do tend to degenerate with age more so than in other parts of the spine, such as the thoracic region. The cervical spine has much greater movement than the mid-back. Where there is greater movement, there is more opportunity for wear and tear on the joints, thus degeneration.

The cervical joints below the axis are capable of various movements including lateral flexion (bending the neck to the side), rotation, and can move dorsally (towards the back) and ventrally (towards the front). Note: The axis is also capable of lateral flexion as well as movements associated with the "No" motion. Each of the neck joints contributes a small amount of movement, but collectively, considerable movement. Chiropractors always strive to maintain normal joint movement, which is why it is important to know which way the joints move.

Thoracic Vertebrae (Mid-Back Bones)

The horse typically has 18 thoracics (dorsals), with few exceptions (the Arabian sometimes has 17). Each thoracic vertebra articulates with a rib on each side, way down deep

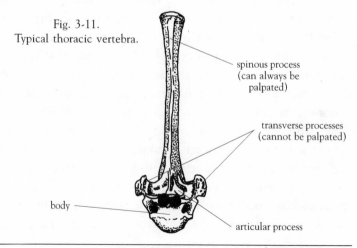

Fig. 3-11.
Typical thoracic vertebra.

spinous process (can always be palpated)

transverse processes (cannot be palpated)

body

articular process

on the transverse processes (see Fig. 3-2). For adjusting purposes, we concern ourselves mainly with the spinouses ("spines") and the angle of the articulating facets and the imbrication of the spines.

The typical thoracic (Fig. 3-11) contains a body, two transverse processes which contain facets for rib attachments, articular processes (facets that articulate one thoracic to another), and a spinous. Of all of these structures, only the tip of the spinouses can be felt and used as adjusting contact points.

The first thoracic is a transition segment from the cervicals; it has a prominent spinous and is often mistaken for the last cervical (see Fig. 3-2). Its spinous is not readily palpable since it is significantly shorter (about half) than the spine of the second dorsal, which can be palpated.

The area of the 3rd through 7th thoracic vertebrae is referred to as the *withers*. This is the highest part of the back below the neck and reaches its summit at the 4th spinous. The withers is also the place where the spines are the longest, thickest, and very palpable (Fig. 3-12). The rest of the thoracics have plate-like spines that too can be easily felt, but not grasped.

An important anatomical consideration in the thoracics is the direction in which the spines point. From the withers to the 15th thoracic, the spines point down towards the tail, or *caudally* (see Fig. 3-2). This direction of the spines is known as *imbrication*, a word often used to describe overlapping shingles of a roof. The 16th thoracic is known as the *anticlinal vertebra*. This vertebra points straight up towards the sky and marks the end of imbrication (see Fig. 3-2). A dog's anticlinal vertebra is the 11th thoracic and often feels

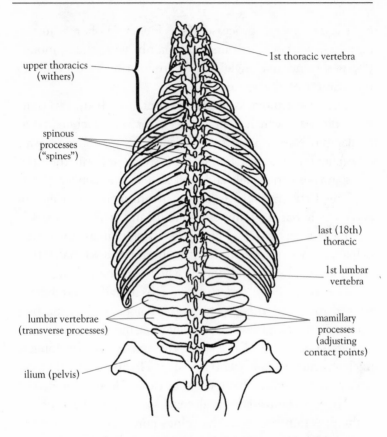

upper thoracics
(withers)

1st thoracic vertebra

spinous
processes
("spines")

last (18th)
thoracic

1st lumbar
vertebra

lumbar vertebrae
(transverse processes)

mamillary
processes
(adjusting
contact points)

ilium (pelvis)

Fig. 3-12. Dorsal (bird's-eye) view of the thoracic and lumbar spine.

like a depression in the back since its spinous is somewhat
smaller than the surrounding spines. A horse's anticlinal
vertebra is always palpable and does not feel like a depression in the back.

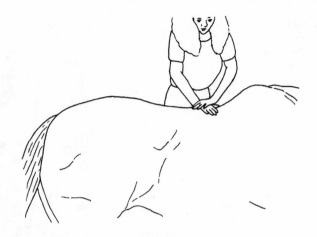

Fig. 3-13. Mid- and lower back adjusting position. Note: The upper thoracics (withers) are not adjusted in this position.

It is essential that you note the direction of the dorsal spinouses. For many of the thoracic adjusting techniques, your thrust/impulse is partially dictated by the direction of the spines. This will be discussed further in the methods sections. But for now, think of your adjusting hand and arm as an extension of the thoracic spines. This is part of the angle of your thrust, impulsing parallel to the grain of the joint facets (Fig. 3-13).

Unlike the 45-degree angle of the cervical zygapophyseal joints, the thoracic articulating surfaces (facets) are in a *coronal plane* (in the direction of the coronal suture of the skull). The best way to imagine a coronal plane is to picture a string tied to the top of your left ear and bringing it over your head to your right ear (Fig. 3-14). Since the thoracic articulating facets mostly face this way, an impulse comple-

Fig. 3-14. Dorsal (top) view of a horse's head, depicting the bones of the skull and the direction of the coronal and sagittal planes.

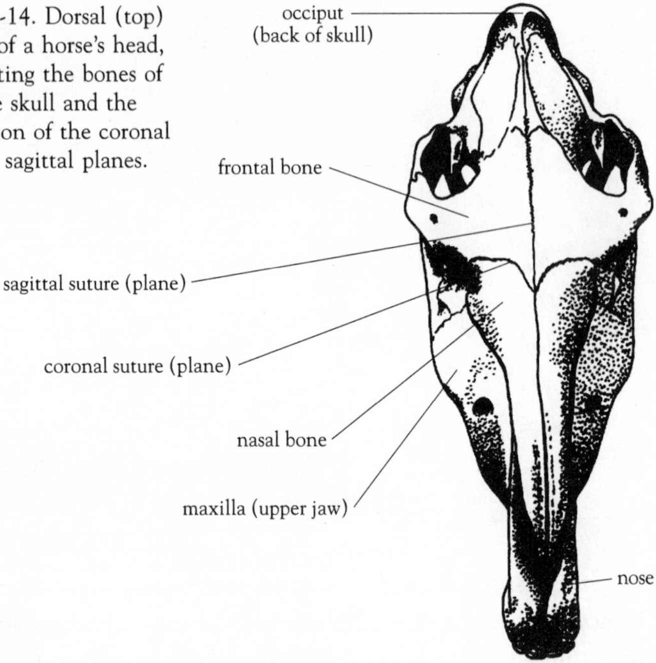

occiput (back of skull)

frontal bone

sagittal suture (plane)

coronal suture (plane)

nasal bone

maxilla (upper jaw)

nose

menting the angles of the spines would also complement the plane line of the facets. This results in a smoother adjustment—going with the flow, if you will, and not jamming the joints. Adjusting against the plane line of the facets would be like stroking your horse's fur the wrong way.

After the 16th thoracic, the remaining two dorsal spines not only point up towards the sky, but a little towards the head as well (cranially)—but only a little. This reversal of sorts is not in sharp contrast to upper thoracic imbrication. While applying an impulse on the lower thoracics and lumbar spinouses,

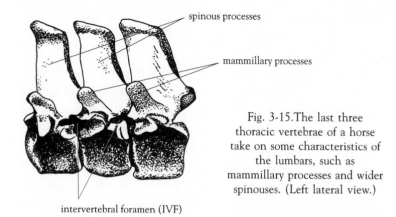

spinous processes

mammillary processes

Fig. 3-15.The last three thoracic vertebrae of a horse take on some characteristics of the lumbars, such as mammillary processes and wider spinouses. (Left lateral view.)

intervertebral foramen (IVF)

you are essentially pushing straight down towards the ground, and only slightly towards the tail (caudally).

The last few thoracics also possess a projection that is indigenous to all of the lumbar vertebrae, mammillary processes. (Fig. 3-15). Though not readily palpable, a mammillary process belonging to the lower thoracics are found on each side of the base of the spinous. On a whole, dry equine skeleton, you can see lower thoracics "transitioning" into the lumbars, taking on some of the lumbar characteristics such as a squatter body and mammillary processes. Just as a reference point, you can always find the last thoracic spine (T18) by feeling the side of the horse, just up from the flank, feeling the last rib and tracing it up as close as you can towards the spine. You will lose your tracing about six inches or so from vertebra T18, since the rib articulates on the transverse process, deep from the spinous. When you lose the rib, simply approximate and continue the curved motion up towards the mid-back.

Nine times out of ten you'll land on T18. For that one time you don't, call Ghostbusters.

Lumbar Vertebrae (Low-Back Bones)

Most horses have six lumbars; Arabians, donkeys, mules, asses, and Przewalski horses sometimes have five. The spines of the lumbars are smaller than those of the thoracics, but are still very palpable. There is a mammillary process projecting up from each side of the *cranial articular processes*, which is roughly on each side of the spinous (Fig. 3-16). The mammillary processes are often used as adjusting contact points. They are situated just forward of its spinous. In other words, as you're scanning down your horse's back (from the withers to the tail), you'll feel the mammillaries first, then scan one more inch towards the tail and you'll feel the spinous of the same vertebra.

The lumbar spinouses make better adjusting contact points only because they're taller than the mammillaries. However, depending on your leverage point during the time of the adjustment, you might want to consider contacting the mammillary. Further explanations are discussed in the method chapters.

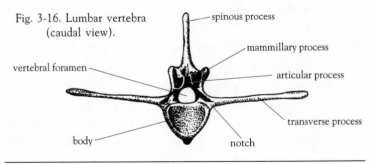

Fig. 3-16. Lumbar vertebra (caudal view).

spinous process

mammillary process

vertebral foramen

articular process

transverse process

body

notch

The lumbar facets (articulating surfaces) differ from those of the dorsals. Their surfaces face sagittally, meaning if you have one on each side, they face each other. To imagine a sagittal plane, just picture a guy with a Mohawk haircut. The center column of hair is in line with the sagittal suture of the skull (see Fig. 3-14). (But the guy with the Mohawk is not in line with society and needs to be adjusted.)

Sacrum

The sacrum is commonly described as one bone, triangular in shape, and consisting of five fused vertebrae (noting occasional exceptions: in the Przewalski horse, Shetland pony, ass, and mule, it can consist of four to six vertebrae). Most

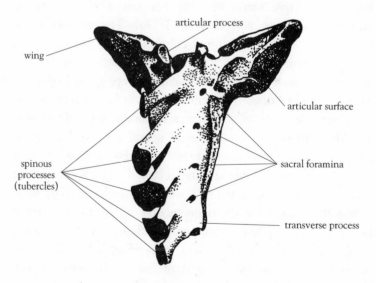

Fig. 3-17. Sacrum of horse (dorso-lateral view).

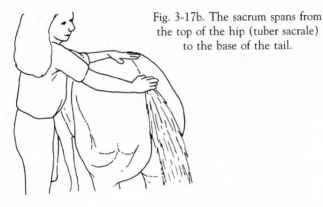

Fig. 3-17b. The sacrum spans from the top of the hip (tuber sacrale) to the base of the tail.

anatomists consider this bone to be part of the spine; it is located directly below the last lumbar, separated by a disc. Each of the five sacral vertebra contains a spinous; these are also known as *tubercles* (Fig. 3-17a). The sacrum is the bone that connects the spinal column to the pelvis.

Equine chiropractors adjust the sacrum quite often. It is an important bone that assists in walking, jumping, and running. In horses, unlike dogs, the sacral spines can be felt quite easily. On either side of the sacral spines exist four dorsal *sacral foramina*, providing an outlet for the sacral spinal nerves. The sacral (cranial) facets which articulate with the last lumbar are in a sagittal ("Mohawk") plane—the left and right surfaces face each other. The sacral wings attach to the ilia (pelvis) with joint surfaces angled at approximately 65 degrees to the vertical (see Fig. 3-17a). These are important adjusting considerations.

We now come to the sacral *apex* (Fig. 3-18). By some accounts, this is the most important area of the spine, period. The sacral apex is located, and can be felt, just above the anus

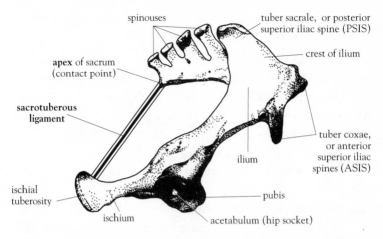

spinouses

tuber sacrale, or posterior superior iliac spine (PSIS)

crest of ilium

apex of sacrum (contact point)

sacrotuberous ligament

tuber coxae, or anterior superior iliac spines (ASIS)

ilium

ischial tuberosity

pubis

ischium

acetabulum (hip socket)

Fig. 3-18. Right hip bone and sacrum of a horse. (Only four out of five spinouses can be seen here, because the first spinous is hidden medially to the tuber sacrale.) The adjusting contact for the Logan Basic Technique is made at the sacral apex. Note: The sacrotuberous ligament is a much broader structure than depicted in this diagram.

as the tail is lifted. There is an important technique called Logan Basic (Ligament Push) that makes use of this point. In fact, there are some equine chiropractors that base their entire technique system around contacting this one point. It is at the apex where an attachment for the *sacrotuberous ligament* can be found and treated. This ligament is not only responsible for several muscular attachments, it can be manipulated in such a way as to affect the hips, spinal cord, and the rest of the vertebral column. You might think of the sacrotuberous ligament as the strings emanating from a hot air balloon basket that connect to the balloon itself, controlling the entire structure by simply tugging on them. This technique is covered in Chapter 13.

Coccygeal Vertebrae (Tail Bones)

The coccygeal or caudal vertebrae number between 15 and 21, with 18 being the average. They reduce in size from the first to the last, where they end up being rod-shaped, the last one having a pointed end. The first two or three tail bones bear articular facets which are directed in the sagittal plane. The tail bones themselves are separated by discs.

Collectively, the tail bones are vital to equine adjusting. These bones are wrapped in muscle and can become gnarled and stiff, and cause back pain as well as dysfunctional locomotion. A tail that is difficult to raise up is a sure sign of back pain. You will see that most tail adjusting methods are traction moves rather than chiropractic adjustments.

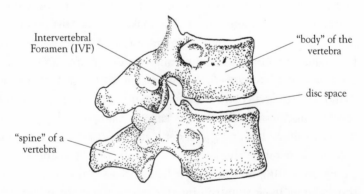

Fig. 3-19. (Right-side view of two human lumbar vertebrae.) The IVF is the opening for a spinal nerve.

Intervertebral Foramen (IVF)

No chiropractic methods book would be complete without discussing the intervertebral foramen, or IVF (Fig. 3-19). This is the primary structure treated by a chiropractor-human patient or otherwise. Simply stated, the IVF is an opening (hole) between two adjacent vertebrae that allows for the passage of a spinal nerve branching from the spinal cord. Other structures contained in the IVF include part of the spinal cord cover (*dura mater*—as in *epidural*, the site of drug injections for pain), the recurrent meningeal nerve (the nerve supply to the disc), intervertebral veins, cerebrospinal fluid, lymphatic vessels, a spinal artery, and connective tissue.

A fixed joint in the spine often means the IVF is less vital, thus encroaching its contents. Chiropractors strive to free up the fixed vertebral joint to restore soft tissue integrity, making its contents vital again. Of the above named structures, the spinal nerve is of central importance. The spinal nerves energize or innervate all of the other components of the body including the skin, muscles and internal organs. Thus, the vertebral subluxation is detrimental to the spinal nerve.

This explanation of the IVF is consistent with standard chiropractic objectives: finding the fixed joint, adjusting it, and ultimately yielding normal nerve expression since the IVF can breathe again. The end result of normal nerve expression is improved organ function and homeostasis (maintaining internal stability). Sounds reasonable. But let's examine this from a practical standpoint. Most conditions equine chiropractors treat have little to do with internal conditions.

They're generally not called out because the horse isn't eating right. Horses are big, physical creatures and are used mainly for strenuous physical activities such as racing, jumping, and pulling. These activities cause stress on the musculoskeletal system, which in turn causes subluxations. By adjusting a subluxation due to physical exertion, we are helping that horse stay physically fit to suit his owner's demands. As a bonus, the owner also gets a horse with improved digestion, breathing, and eliminating systems. This is sort of chiropractic philosophy in reverse—but it works!

We know that tight muscles and ligaments can squeeze the spine, crowding the contents of the IVF and thereby blunting the nerve signals. The intended organ or muscle doesn't gets a full blast of power. It's the difference between hearing a knock on the door loud and clear when you're in the living room, or barely hearing it in the bedroom.

An encroachment of a single spinal nerve can affect one's overall health. For example, if the spinal nerve leading to the stomach is subluxated, digestion might become disrupted due to abnor-

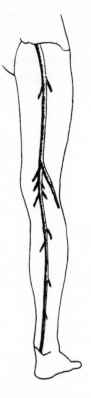

Fig. 3-20. Human sciatic nerve—the large nerve of the leg. This nerve can become pinched along its course, but is often irritated where it originates: in the lumbar region of the spine.

mal gastric juice production. If any one system in the body is malfunctioning, it puts a strain on the rest of the body, creating even more subluxations and/or compensations. This is why regular chiropractic checkups are necessary: to catch and treat subluxations before they fester into a crisis.

The urgency of keeping the IVF open and biomechanically sound doesn't become apparent to most people unless they experience severe pain, as with sciatica or pain down the leg (Fig. 3-20). The sciatic nerve, which is the thickest nerve in the human body, originates from the lower spinal nerves and branches down, supplying the legs with sensory and motor functions. Often, sciatica is caused by an encroachment of the spinal nerve as it leaves the spinal column at the IVF. This encroachment can be caused by a variety of irritating factors, including tight spinal muscles (spasms), joint degeneration, or a herniated disc. Orthopedic surgeons perform operations that are designed to make sure the IVF is clear. One such operation is called a *laminectomy*. This procedure restores the natural opening of the IVF by removing some of the diseased bone tissue (usually caused by arthritic buildup surrounding the lamina) which was blocking that space where the spinal nerve exits. Another operation is called a *discectomy*. Here, the surgeon removes part or all of a bulging disc which was also creating a barrier and pressure on the spinal nerve. In each case, these surgeries are necessary—and more often than not, successful—for relieving pain and restoring proper function of the sciatic nerve. **Note:** Chiropractors can also successfully treat sciatica if it is due to nerve pressure caused by muscle spasms constricting the spine. But when there is a mechanical blockage, such as a herniated disc, surgery is usually the most effective and permanent treatment.

This example of IVF encroachment describes a crisis situation. The subluxation, however, is much more subtle since pain isn't always involved. Spinal subluxations are of epidemic proportions in both man and beast, and if left untreated, they will eventually cause dis-ease. *The significance of the IVF cannot be overstated.* The explanation above demonstrates how two professions (orthopedic surgeons and chiropractors) both make a living out of keeping the IVF clear.

Hips (Pelvic Bones)

The pelvis is a large, bony apparatus consisting of three major components, the *ischium*, *ilium*, and *pubis*, and serves to connect the spine to the body via the *sacroiliac* joint (see Fig. 3-18). The pelvis is a prime example of a colossal part of the horse that seems impossible to adjust by hand. Yet as massive as the pelvis is, it has a few strategically placed bony levers that can be used by the practitioner to deliver a smooth, though not entirely effortless, adjustment.

I won't lie to you. You do have to have some physical attributes to adjust a horse by hand. I would agree with most chiropractors that speed is the key element necessary to deliver a safe and effective adjustment, but it also doesn't hurt if you weigh over 150 pounds and have ample biceps. This is not to say that a slight person cannot adjust a horse. They certainly can. But they need to compensate for their lack of size by developing lightning-fast arm and chest muscle actions. The same can be said for the five-foot, 102-pound

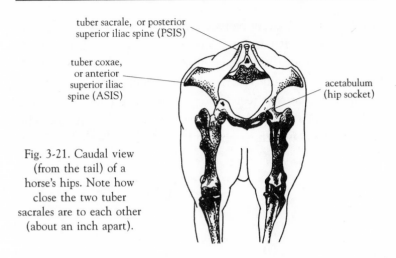

tuber sacrale, or posterior superior iliac spine (PSIS)

tuber coxae, or anterior superior iliac spine (ASIS)

acetabulum (hip socket)

Fig. 3-21. Caudal view (from the tail) of a horse's hips. Note how close the two tuber sacrales are to each other (about an inch apart).

man who wants to flip a six-foot-five, 240-pound man in his judo class. With the right technique, he can do it.

The pelvis is the foundation of the body where powerful muscles as well as the hind limbs attach. There are basically three points of the pelvis that are regularly used in the practice of equine chiropractic: the tuber sacrale (posterior-superior-iliac-spine or PSIS), the tuber coxae (anterior-superior-iliac-spine or ASIS), and the acetabulum or hip socket (Fig. 3-21).

The PSIS or tuber sacrales are the highest points of the pelvis and are used to adjust the sacroiliac joints. They are called the tuber sacrales because of their proximity to the sacrum. From Fig. 3-21 you can see there are two tubers, one on top of each ilium. These are the "magic" points of hip adjusting. Knowing how to feel and contact these two spots will enable you to adjust even the biggest draft horse's pelvis.

Luckily, they're easily palpated, but they are deceptively close to each other. If you firmly run your thumb and index finger on each side of the lumbar spine and scan towards the rump, you will eventually reach a bony summit (Fig. 3-22). This summit will at first feel like one bone, but if you pierce the center of this hill with your finger, you'll feel a crevice. This crevice separates the right and left PSIS's. Both PSIS's are

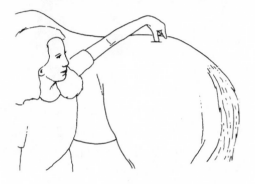

Fig. 3-22. Touching the PSIS's (tuber sacrales).

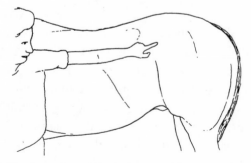

Fig. 3-23. Touching the ASIS's (tuber coxae), a.k.a. the point of the hip—an important adjusting point.

confined to a six- to eight-inch circumference. **Important anatomical landmark:** Directly below the crevice mentioned above is the first sacral tubercle (spine). The entire sacrum can be palpated from that point all the way to the base of the tail. No part of the sacrum is cranial (forward) of the PSIS.

The ASIS or tuber coxae are large bony masses that can be felt at the side of the horse's rump. They literally "stick out" as you feel your way across the side of the pelvis. The ASIS is considered the "point" of the hip (Fig. 3-23). Most people are tall enough to contact and adjust this point by simply standing next to their horse. The ASIS is often used to adjust the hip when a PSIS contact is too awkward to use— namely, in situations where an assistant refuses to extend the hind leg, which aids in the PSIS adjustment (see Chapter 14).

The acetabulum or hip socket (Fig. 3-24) is formed by the junction of the ilium, pubis, and ischium. The ball or head of the femur (thigh bone) fits into this socket to form

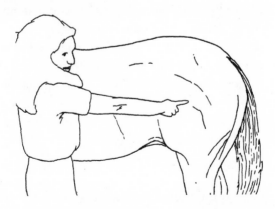

Fig. 3-24. Touching the hip socket (see also Fig. 3-18).

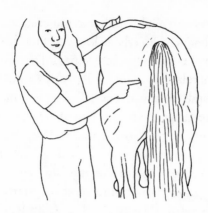

Fig. 3-25. Touching the ischium, which is part of the hip (see Fig. 3-18), but not recommended as an adjusting point.

the hip joint. Often the soundness of this joint is a measure of how the entire pelvis, lower back, and hind limbs are functioning. Stress here can affect the entire musculoskeletal system.

The other parts of the pelvis are also important, but are seldom used as adjusting points. The *ischium*, for example, is an important muscular and ligamentous attachment site and looks like a good lever, but it is dangerous to contact since a push here can disconcert the horse and cause him to kick (Fig. 3-25). The *pubis* is also an important muscular attachment site, but difficult to contact. Incidentally, the pelvis and associated structures are markedly bigger in the mare compared to the stallion, to make it easier to give birth.

The Head

Discussing the horse's head at this point is like putting the cart before the—well, you know. But the truth of the matter is that the movement of the horse's head along with its neck plays a crucial role during running and jumping.

In Chapter 11 you will learn methods to adjust your horse's neck in relation to the base of the skull (occiput), and later, methods to adjust the only freely moveable joint in the head, the *temporomandibular joint* or TMJ. The TMJ is

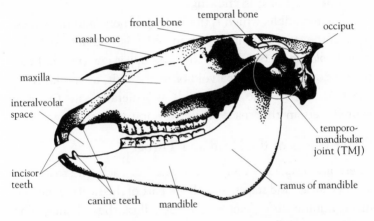

Fig. 3-26. Left side of horse skull. Note the temporomandibular joint (TMJ).

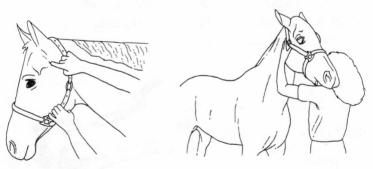

Fig. 3-27a. Touching the TMJ. Fig. 3-27b. Palpating both TMJ's.

a joint formed between the *ramus* of the *mandible* and the *temporal* bone on either side (Fig. 3-26). It is a powerful hinge and gliding joint which often subluxates in response to improperly fitting bits, riders tugging too hard on the reins, and above all, atlas misalignments. Its movement can be felt by placing your hands at the area pictured in Fig. 3-27 while the horse is chewing.

The mandible, which is the lower jaw bone and the largest bone of the face, contains a section which is void of teeth—the *interalveolar space* (see Fig. 3-26). The upper jaw (*maxilla*) features a corresponding area void of teeth. This, as you know, is the space where the bit goes. It is generally safe to place your fingers in this space while working with the jaw.

Other Bones of the Head and Throat

There are 3 *auditory ossicles* contained in each inner ear, the *malleus*, *incus*, and *stapes*, and all are part of the hearing mechanism. Equine chiropractors do not adjust these bones. The ossicles are difficult to feel (if not impossible) and they rarely malfunction, except during those times when the horse completely ignores you while you're shouting, "Get off my foot, you big lummox!"

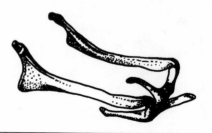

Fig. 3-28. The hyoid bone, a bone in the throat. (Rostrolateral view—from the right side.)

The *hyoid bone* is a strange-looking structure composed of many parts, which is situated just under the mandible (Fig. 3-28). It attaches to several structures including the tongue, the pharynx, and the larynx. The pharynx is the tube or cavity, with its surrounding membrane and muscles, that connects the mouth and nasal passages with the esophagus. The larynx is the site of the vocal cords. A hoarse horse may have an inflamed larynx, or a horse who has trouble swallowing may have an inflamed pharynx. In either case, gentle manipulation (tugging and rocking) of the hyoid bone would help relieve soft-tissue stress in the throat.

Clavicle (Collarbone)

There is none. A collarbone would restrict the horse's running ability, since a full shoulder girdle complete with a clavicle would inhibit scapular movements, thus limiting the foreleg swing. And while we're at it, horses don't have a gallbladder either. This is most likely due to their naturally low-fat diet.

Sternum (Breastbone)

The *sternum* (breastbone) is a flat, canoe-shaped bone comprised of 6 to 8 bony segments (sternebrae) that are connected to each other by cartilage (Fig. 3-29). The first 8 pairs of ribs articulate with the sternum. The sternum forms the floor of the thoracic cavity. Labored breathing may be due to a restriction of the costal (rib) joints. Light to moderate pressure applied over the rib joints here often facilitates chest expansion, thus making breathing easier.

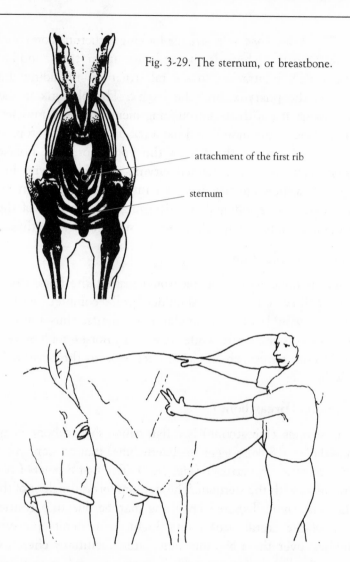

Fig. 3-29. The sternum, or breastbone.

attachment of the first rib

sternum

Fig. 3-30. Touching the scapula, or shoulder blade (see also Fig. 3-2).

Scapula (Shoulder Bone)

The scapula is a flat bone whose top borders (which are cartilaginous) span the second to seventh dorsal spines. It articulates with the humerus, but does not form a true shoulder joint since there is no clavicle. The scapula provides surfaces for important muscular attachments. Tight or stressed scapular muscles are often eased all at once with a proper adjustment, affording immediate relief to the shoulder and forelimb. Take note of the spine of the scapula; this easily palpable anatomical landmark will help you feel the rest of the bone. When you run your hands along the side of the shoulder (Fig. 3-30), the scapular spine will feel like a hard vertical bony ridge. It is the only vertical ridge in that area, unlike a curved rib.

The Foreleg

The bones of the foreleg (thoracic limb), along with its muscles, tendons and ligaments, constitute an impressive structure that not only must support over 60 percent of the horse's weight, but the rider's as well. Aside from being a weight-bearing extremity, the thoracic limb also works as the body's steering wheel.

A series of ingeniously arranged bones and joints is the makeup of this marvel of engineering. In essence, the bones and joints of the forelimb are designed to absorb shock when the foot strikes the ground, and afford enough flexibility in the event of sudden stops and while negotiating changing terrain.

The leg's shock-absorbing ability is greatly due to the curved or bowed nature of the bones themselves. When you look at most of the long bones of the foreleg (Fig. 3-31a), you can see

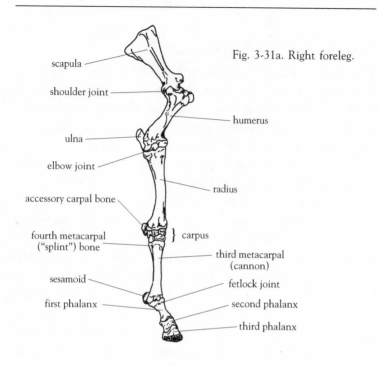

Fig. 3-31a. Right foreleg.

scapula

shoulder joint

humerus

ulna

elbow joint

radius

accessory carpal bone

fourth metacarpal ("splint") bone

carpus

third metacarpal (cannon)

sesamoid

fetlock joint

first phalanx

second phalanx

third phalanx

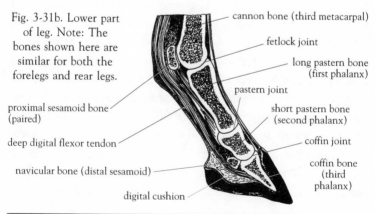

Fig. 3-31b. Lower part of leg. Note: The bones shown here are similar for both the forelegs and rear legs.

cannon bone (third metacarpal)

fetlock joint

long pastern bone (first phalanx)

pastern joint

short pastern bone (second phalanx)

proximal sesamoid bone (paired)

deep digital flexor tendon

coffin joint

navicular bone (distal sesamoid)

coffin bone (third phalanx)

digital cushion

either a pronounced curve, as in the *radius*, or a subtle curve, as in the third metacarpal bone (*cannon bone*). A bowed stick will displace shock more efficiently than a straight one. For example, if you break your leg, you may be forced to walk with a cane for a while until you heal. If you're like most people, you'll buy a cane at your local pharmacy. But what does your local pharmacy sell you? A cane which is essentially a straight, hard stick that has no give and shakes when it strikes the ground, causing your fracture to vibrate with pain. Nothing could be more unlike your own leg. What you should be using is one of nature's canes such as a sassafras root—the kind you find stacked next to the umbrellas in a "historical" cave's souvenir shop near the Smokies (although I don't think Geronimo cared much for Brach's™ Maple-Nut Goodies).

From Fig. 3-31a, you'll discover that a horse's forelegs are very similar to our own thoracic limbs, the arms. We both have shoulder blades (*scapulas*), as well as a *humerus* in each foreleg (upper arm bones). Our forearm bones differ slightly from an equine's. We both have a *radius* and *ulna*, but a horse's ulna is reduced and partially lost, mainly representing the point of the elbow (*olecranon process*). The lower end of the ulna is fused with the radius, forming part of the joint that articulates with the first row of *carpal* bones (the wrist or knee). The horse's carpal bones or *carpus* are equivalent to our wrist; this group of bones and joints is commonly referred to as the knee, but does not correspond to the human knee.

Below the carpus (knee), there are some notable differences between man and horse. We have five fingers, but a horse has one main "finger" and two smaller or reduced ones.

Horses don't have a thumb or a little finger. The *splint bones* (*second metacarpals*) are roughly similar to our ring and index fingers. Our middle finger is ostentatiously represented as the horse's long and strong *third metacarpal* or *cannon bone*. The *fetlock* joint or knuckle, which is the so-called "ankle" of the horse (not corresponding to our ankle), is formed by the cannon bone articulating with the upper end of the *long pastern bone*—

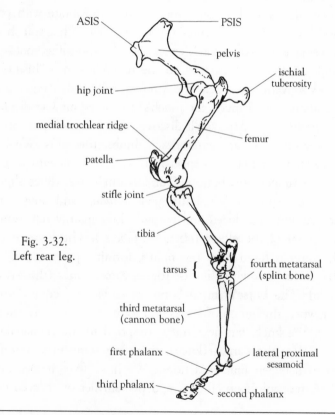

ASIS

PSIS

pelvis

ischial tuberosity

hip joint

medial trochlear ridge

femur

patella

stifle joint

tibia

Fig. 3-32. Left rear leg.

tarsus {

fourth metatarsal (splint bone)

third metatarsal (cannon bone)

first phalanx

lateral proximal sesamoid

third phalanx

second phalanx

the first *phalanx*. A phalanx is roughly the same as a finger or toe. The first phalanx joins the shorter second phalanx, which joins with the third phalanx (*coffin bone* or *pedal bone*). There is a clinically significant bone called the *navicular bone* (a.k.a. the *distal sesamoid*) located on the back side (above the "heel"), between the second phalanx (*short pastern*) and the third phalanx. The navicular bone is found both in the forelegs and rear legs, but is most often associated with lameness in the foreleg.

The Rear Leg

There are more similarities than differences between the forelegs and rear legs (Fig. 3-32). The scapula would approximately correspond to the *femur* (thigh bone; the top aspect of the femur, the *greater trochanter*, is known as the *whorlbone*); the humerus would compare to the *tibia* (shinbone), the elbow would relate to the *hock* (the ankle and heel equivalent in a person), and the rear cannon would equal the sum of the radius, knee, and cannon of the foreleg. This is because the *tarsal bones* (hock) of the rear legs do not replicate the more independent movements of the carpus. In fact, the fetlock, hock, and *stifle* (which is the true knee formed by the articulation of the femur and tibia—complete with a *patella* or kneecap) cannot flex independently of each other. For your convenience, however, everything below the hock is the same as on the foreleg.

The Stay Mechanism

The horse has a rather intriguing ability—to remain standing while sleeping. This is made possible by the *stay mechanism*. This structural phenomenon is accomplished though a series of intricate ligamentous and muscular pulls which stabilizes both the fore- and hind legs while at rest. These muscles and ligaments lock the key joints in the "stay" position. There is a complicated and dizzying explanation of how this works. In part, there is a locking device at the stifle (the joint corresponding to the human knee). When the hind leg is extended, the patella (kneecap) can be pulled sideways and hooked over an enlarged prominence of the femur (thighbone) called the *medial trochlear ridge* (see Fig. 3-32). The horse can free himself from this position by simply contracting a couple of thigh muscles (*quadriceps* and the *tensor fasciae latae*), thus unlocking the patella by lifting it up and over the ridge, which frees the stifle and allows the horse to move again. However, the stay mechanism is only effective during the more shallow *slow-wave* sleep. During the deeper *paradoxical sleep* (a.k.a. rapid-eye-movement sleep), a horse must be recumbent.

The Muscles

You cannot be a complete equine chiropractor if you think your job is to simply move bones. The fact is, the muscles constitute approximately 60 percent of the horse's body weight. They can't be ignored. The equine chiropractor frequently has to wade through bulky muscle mass to reach the bony contact points. Volumes have been written on the equine muscular system and ways to treat it. While this book is technically not about treating muscles, it is important that you have at least a working knowledge of the muscular system and some of the muscle therapies that complement the chiropractic adjustment.

What Is A Muscle?

The Random House dictionary defines *muscle* as "a tissue composed of cells or fibers, the contraction of which produces movement in the body." A more precise chiropractic definition would read: Muscles are soft fibrous tissues that contract and produce body movements *when energized by nerve impulses*. Muscles also give the body bulk and shape, and can become knotted in response to sudden movements.

There are three types of muscles in the body: *smooth muscles*, found in the blood vessels and hollow organs; *cardiac muscles*, found only in the heart; and *skeletal muscles* (a.k.a. voluntary muscles—numbering about 700 in the horse) which attach to the bones and account for more than half of the horse's body weight. Wherever you see a reference to muscles in this book, we're discussing skeletal muscles. All areas of your horse's body (except the lower legs—below the carpus or tarsus) are covered by skeletal muscles ranging in size from the very minute eye muscles to the bulky rump muscles. In those lower-leg areas that are devoid of muscle tissue, the upper-leg muscles "stretch" their tendons down the leg and over the joints. These tendons are protected by sheaths, or tendon *bursae* (sacs).

Muscles are able to perform work because they are attached to bones by tendons. There are generally two places a muscle attaches to a bone: the *origin* or more fixed point; and the *insertion*, the more moveable point, found further down the bone. When massage therapists work on your body, they concentrate on one or two muscles at a time in a particular area in order to free them up. When chiropractors adjust a bone, they are able to influence all of the muscles originating and inserting from that particular bone—all at once. This is why an adjustment is such an efficient treatment. A full spine/ body adjustment requires only a fraction of the time it takes to perform a full-body massage.

You can think of the musculoskeletal system as a series of puppets in a marionette show: the bones are the puppets and the muscles are the strings. The puppets would not be able to move in any meaningful way if the strings were not attached in strategic areas. This is precisely the relationship the bones have with the muscles, making up a series of levers, pulleys and cables. This is also the basis for spotting lameness.

When you suffer a sprained neck, the first thing you notice is pain, because your neck is restricted. One of the strings is too tight and can't do its job. But this isn't all bad. Your body doesn't give you anything you don't need. A muscle spasm is simply a natural body splint that stops your body from moving in order to prevent further injury. People who pay attention to this warning signal and stop lifting weights for a week will mend faster. In this sense, horses are smarter than people. When a horse suffers a severe muscle cramp, it will try to stand still or lie down for a while and let its muscle heal, since it doesn't fear getting fired for skipping work. No competent trainer would work a horse past the point of pain.

The bones are a series of levers that are moved by muscles. Proper movement of joints is produced by muscles working in harmony. When your body is in motion, some muscles relax while others contract. A muscle that is stretched or massaged before an athletic event is less likely to sustain injury because

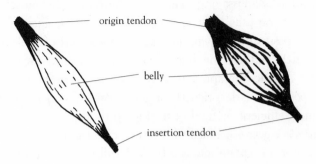

Fig. 3-33a. Relaxed muscle.　　　Fig. 3-33b. Contracted muscle.

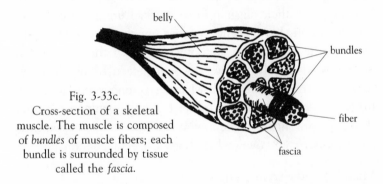

Fig. 3-33c.
Cross-section of a skeletal
muscle. The muscle is composed
of *bundles* of muscle fibers; each
bundle is surrounded by tissue
called the *fascia*.

it can adapt to sudden movements better than a stiff muscle. In other words, the muscle "has already been there."

The various types of muscle therapies are identified by the part of the muscle that is treated. *Trigger point therapy*, for example, is a technique requiring the therapist to apply pressure in the center or *belly* of the muscle (Figs. 3-33a–c) in order to clean out and release toxins. *Transverse Friction Massage* (TFM) is also a technique used to clean out a muscle and break up adhesions by massaging against the grain of the muscle. A muscle therapy called the *Origin-Insertion Technique* releases muscle spasms by applying pressure to both ends of the muscle (tendons)–"pulling the hammock at both ends." Of all the equine muscle therapies, it is my opinion that treating the *stress points* (muscle origins), or *Stress Point Therapy* (SPT), is the most efficient method of freeing up the limb with immediate needs–e.g., for a horse who has to race the next day. Since this is not an equine massage book, I will primarily discuss the superficial muscles which you'll need to know in order to apply SPT. Superficial muscles are muscles you can "get at" with your fingers without digging for bedrock. During the course of this discussion, I will mention other muscles and their importance in the body. Note: The order in which the muscles will be discussed closely follows the sequence used by world-renowned sports therapist Jack Meagher (pronounced "Mar") in his book *Beating Muscle Injuries For Horses*. I highly recommend this book for horse owners who are serious about winning more races or improving their horse's overall performance.

Muscles and Stress Points

There's no sense in reinventing the wheel here, so I'm not going to name the muscle origins and insertions except in a general way. If you must know this information, refer to Sisson and Grossman's *Anatomy of the Domestic Animals* (see bibliography). By looking at Figs. 3-34 through 3-37, you'll get a good idea where these muscles are with accordance to your immediate needs. For example, if your horse can't walk a straight line and is off on circles, you'll know it's a problem with the *brachio-*

cephalicus muscle. The diagrams show you where the muscles are; Fig. 3-38 shows the stress points, which are the areas where you apply pressure to help the problem. Note: Stress points are found at the *origin* of the muscle, where the muscle is anchored to the bone and has less mobility. For each stress area treated, apply light to moderate pressure for 3–5 minutes. Study the following list of muscles to help you isolate and treat the appropriate areas (the numbers correspond to Fig. 3-38).

1. **Rectus capitus lateralis:** This muscle helps bend the top of the neck down (flexion of the first two cervical vertebrae). If your horse makes continuous stretching movements with his head and carries his head low to one side, consider treating the stress point and adjusting either the atlas or axis.

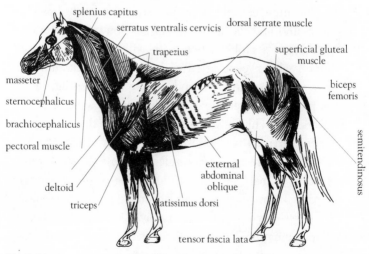

Fig. 3-34.

2. **Brachiocephalicus:** This muscle wears many hats; it helps extend (raise up) the shoulder, head, and neck, assists in moving the head and neck to the side, and also serves to move the foreleg. If your horse has difficulty walking a straight line and is off on circles, treat the stress point here and look for a subluxation at the 7th cervical.

3. **Multifidus cervicus:** Besides flexing the neck to one side, this muscle rotates the head to the opposite side. If your horse has a problem here, you'll notice he resists turning his neck to the opposite side of the muscle. Look for a lower cervical subluxation.

4. **Rhomboidius:** These are actually two muscles, one named after the neck (*rhomboidius cervicus*) and the other for the top of the mid-back (*rhomboidius thoracis*). These muscles help draw the shoulder blade upward (dorsally) and forward (cranially, or towards the head). If there is a problem here, you will notice your horse flinch when you touch his shoulders, exhibit difficulties with coordination, and display a non-specific loss of power. A lower cervical subluxation may be present.

5. **Trapezius:** This muscle is also named for the neck (*trapezius cervicus*) and mid-back (*trapezius thoracis*). The problems here are very similar to those of the rhomboidius, namely, generalized tightening of the shoulders (spasms), loss of power, and decreased neck flexibility. A lower cervical subluxation may also be present here.

6. **Supraspinatus:** This muscle extends (opens) the shoulder joint and helps prevent dislocation of the shoulder.

If there is pain here, your horse will bend his knees in response to firm pressure over this muscle. Again, a lower cervical subluxation can be noticed.

7. **Infraspinatus:** This muscle also helps to support the shoulder to prevent dislocation; it also abducts

Fig. 3-35.

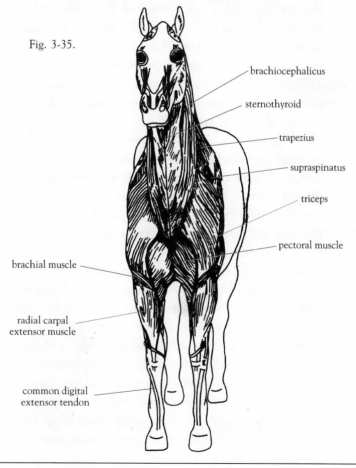

brachiocephalicus

sternothyroid

trapezius

supraspinatus

triceps

pectoral muscle

brachial muscle

radial carpal
extensor muscle

common digital
extensor tendon

the foreleg (moves the foreleg *away* from the body) and rotates the foreleg outward. Problems with this muscle are similar to those of the supraspinatus.

8. **Serratus thoracics:** This muscle helps support the trunk when the leg is planted on the ground; it also moves the scapula back towards the tail (caudally). When this muscle is stressed, you might notice the saddle slipping off to one side. This often coincides with a mid- to lower cervical subluxation.

9. **Triceps (upper end):** This part of the triceps flexes the shoulder joint. Trouble here may result in a shortened foreleg stride, as well as looking lame at extended trot. If this is the case, look for a lower cervical or upper thoracic subluxation.

10. **Triceps (lower end):** This muscle extends and locks the elbow joint. If this muscle was affected, you might see a shortened stride, as well as your horse avoiding the lead when jumping. A lower cervical or upper thoracic subluxation may be partially to blame.

11. **Pectoralis:** This muscle and its divisions draw the front leg backwards as well as advancing the leg. A problem here may result in a short extension of the forelimb; your horse may refuse to take proper leads and/or show discomfort while tightening the girth. Look for a lower cervical and an upper thoracic subluxation.

12. **Longissmus dorsi:** This is a powerful extensor on the back and also assists in lateral flexion of the spine. When injured, this muscle is often involved in back pain, loss of coordinated power while in motion, and

the site of the "cold back." Jumpers often stress this muscle due to jarring upon landing. Nerves from various vertebral levels supply this muscle area, including nerves from the cervical, thoracic and lumbar regions. Therefore, check all spinal levels if this muscle is stressed.

Fig. 3-36.

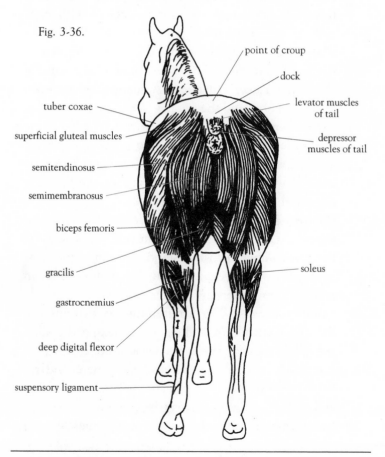

point of croup

dock

levator muscles of tail

tuber coxae

depressor muscles of tail

superficial gluteal muscles

semitendinosus

semimembranosus

biceps femoris

gracilis

soleus

gastrocnemius

deep digital flexor

suspensory ligament

13. **Longissimus costarum:** This muscle assists in lateral flexion of the trunk. When stressed, the longissmus costarum will restrict lateral bending of the trunk. Look for thoracic and lumbar subluxations.

14. **Gluteus medius:** Aside from extending the hip, the gluteus medius moves the hindlimb outward. This muscle is frequently the area associated with back pain, a shortened stride, and restricting hip extension. It is also closely involved with the actions of the longissmus dorsi. This is the muscle that will dip or sag upon deep palpation. A subluxation between the 6th lumbar and the sacrum can affect this muscle.

15. **Biceps femoris:** This muscle is used to extend the hip, stifle, hock and rear leg, and is also for rear leg propulsion. Stress at this muscle can lead to shortened forward movement. Subluxations often occurring at the lower lumbar region.

16. **Gastrocnemius:** This muscle extends the hock and flexes the stifle. Stress at this muscle can make the horse uncomfortable while standing, or may not allow his stifle to straighten. Lower lumbar subluxations can be found here when this muscle is stressed.

17. **Semitendinosus:** The semitendinosus extends the hip and hock joints, and assists in flexing the stifle as well as rotating the lower leg inward. Stress here can result in shortened forward movement and resisting the stifle to be straightened. Lower lumbar and sacral subluxations may be present.

18. **Semimembranosus:** The action of this muscle is to

extend the hip joint and draw the lower leg inward (adduction). A problem with this muscle can be seen as a shortened forward stride, resisting lateral movement, and refusal to straighten the stifle. Upon firm palpation of this muscle, the lower leg may react by tucking in. Look for lower lumbar and upper sacral subluxations.

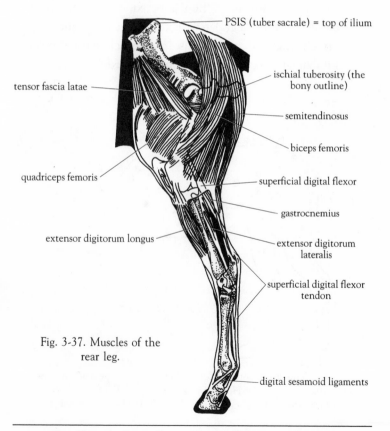

PSIS (tuber sacrale) = top of ilium

ischial tuberosity (the bony outline)

tensor fascia latae

semitendinosus

biceps femoris

quadriceps femoris

superficial digital flexor

gastrocnemius

extensor digitorum longus

extensor digitorum lateralis

superficial digital flexor tendon

Fig. 3-37. Muscles of the rear leg.

digital sesamoid ligaments

19. **Tensor fascia lata:** This muscle flexes the hip joint and extends the stifle. If this muscle is stressed, the horse may throw his rear limb outward on the forward stride, as well as restricting lateral movements. Lower lumbar and upper sacral subluxations may cause the above problems.

20. **Illiacus:** This muscle flexes the hip joint and rotates the thigh outward. When affected, this muscle may cause the hind leg(s) to buckle, can cause stumbling on circles, and appears as lower back pain. Lower lumbar subluxations may be involved.

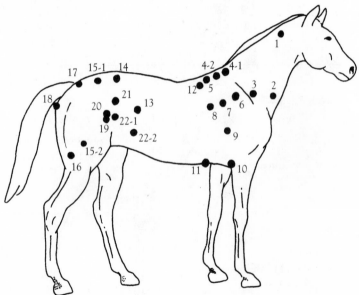

Fig. 3-38. The stress points. Note: These points appear in the book *Beating Muscle Injuries for Horses* by Jack Meagher. (The numbers of the points shown here vary slightly from Mr. Meagher's book.)

21. **Gluteus accessorius:** Aside from assisting the gluteus muscle in extending the hip, this muscle rotates the thigh outward. Stress here may cause back pain, restricted hip movement and a shorted forward stride. Lower lumbar and sacral subluxations may be involved.

22. **External oblique:** This muscle flexes the trunk. A problem here can affect lateral movements and may be associated with "tying-up," which is a term used to describe a form of *azoturia*. With azoturia, excessive amounts of nitrogen waste products are found in the urine, caused by the excessive breakdown of muscle tissue. Kidney failure may result if this condition isn't properly treated. Look for lower lumbar subluxations.

Now that you've been exposed to the workings of the horse's musculoskeletal system, you should be familiar with some of the more common conditions affecting bones and muscles. These conditions must be ruled out before adjusting your horse, since some of them cannot effectively be treated with chiropractic care. (The next chapter will explain further.)

NERVES

As detailed in Appendix B (p. 287), it was a condition caused by a pinched nerve that gave chiropractic its start. In 1895, a janitor named Harvey Lillard complaining of hearing loss sought the help of Dr. Daniel David Palmer, a magnetic healer who practiced in Davenport, Iowa. Mr. Lillard told Dr. Palmer that he had injured his back seventeen years earlier, and had had diminished hearing ever since. When Dr. Palmer examined Mr. Lillard's spine, he felt a misaligned vertebra, and proceeded to "rack it" into place (after which Dr. Palmer probably experienced some hearing loss of his own). This was the first chiropractic adjustment—and it restored Mr. Lillard's hearing.

Whether or not the above story is based on 100 percent fact, the world may never know. But the truth is, nerves are

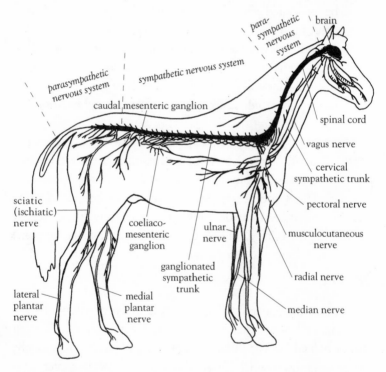

Fig. 3-39. The nervous system. The shaded areas (brain and spinal cord) make up the central nervous system. The peripheral nervous system consists of all the other nerves.

everywhere in the body, and their connections are widespread. It is entirely possible that a pinched spinal nerve can affect hearing. The chiropractic subluxation theory is based on the fact that spinal nerves can be pinched between the vertebrae and that this causes distress to the related muscle or organ.

The nervous system is divided into two parts: the *central nervous system*, which includes your brain and spinal cord, and the *peripheral nervous system*, which includes everything else (Fig. 3-39). The spinal nerves are part of the peripheral nervous system, and the spine is the area most often treated by chiropractors for pinched nerves. The spine is the switchboard of the body. Every neurological transmission, whether coming from the body to the brain (*afferent pathways*) or from the brain to the body (*efferent pathways*), must pass through the spine. A blockage of these signals will impair body-to-brain communication and cause disease. Chiropractic strives to maintain body communication.

There is frequently a confusion of terms relating to the back, especially the differences between the *spinal cord*, the *spinal column*, and *spinal nerves*. The spinal cord is nerve tissue protected within the spinal column (back bones or vertebrae), much as the brain is protected by the skull. Spinal nerves are long nerves that originate in the spinal cord and pass through openings in the spinal column, making their way to the rest of the body.

The part of the peripheral nervous system over which you have little or no control is called the *autonomic nervous system*. The "autonomics," also referred to as the *involuntary* and/or *vegetative* nervous system, control your breathing while you sleep, your heart rate, and your glandular functions, to name a few. The part of the nervous system is particularly important because your horse may not show any signs of distress; conditions of the autonomics are mostly silent until they culminate into a crisis in the form of muscle spasms or internal dis-ease. This is why you must always check your horse's spine for subluxations. Stop problems before they happen. Practice maintenance care.

For those concerned mostly about lameness in their horse (problems with the gait), you should know that the spinal nerves located at the upper part of your horse's back control his front legs. The low-back spinal nerves control his hind legs. The mid-back spinal nerves control the surrounding muscles. Almost the entire range of spinal nerves regulates the internal organs in some way.

You cannot feel pinched nerves, but you can make an educated guess about their specific locations by knowing what ails your horse. If your vet has diagnosed a stomach condition, look for areas on the spine that relate to the stomach (see Fig. 17-1). You'll also learn from the examination chapter that true subluxations or pinched spinal nerves have a few things in common. Some of the most common signs of vertebral subluxations include restricted joint motion over the painful area, a hard muscle knot next to a "spine," and increased heat on that hard knot.

For those less experienced with examining horses, the first thing you'll notice is that a horse feels warmer. A healthy horse's temperature is about 99.5˚–100.5˚F (compared to 98.6˚F for people). Get used to feeling the warmth of the whole horse before you start isolating prospective trouble spots. It takes experience and a sensitive touch to distinguish warm spots from hot spots, mainly because the hair/coat is a barrier to the skin.

CHAPTER 4

PALPATION
(FEELING FOR SUBLUXATIONS)

Palpation is a skill in and of itself. Anyone can walk up to a horse and start crackin' away. However, that's not chiropractic. Moving those bones in an arbitrary way may constitute a form of Stalin-era torture, but since your horse will never give up the secret rocket fuel formula, you might as well adjust only those joints that need fixing.

There are two basic palpation skills: *static palpation* and *motion palpation*. Both of these skills should be attempted only after a thorough gait analysis (see Chapter 6). I generally start with static palpation immediately following the gait analysis. Note: It is imperative that you fully absorb Chapter 3 before you can appreciate palpation.

STATIC PALPATION

The whole idea of static palpation is to feel your horse while he's standing still in a neutral position, and as relaxed as possible. He has to be relaxed because when you feel a bone or joint, you're actually testing its resistance in relation to the immediate structures, such as the bones above and below, as well as the surrounding muscles. For example, any movement of his head while you're palpating his neck will change your entire analysis. Also, you don't need to have your horse artificially relaxed with medications. Unnatural relaxants such as tranquilizers will also alter your analysis. Tranquilizers, however, do come in handy when it's time to adjust a rambunctious patient. Since each part of the body relates to the whole, I will discuss not only spinal palpation, but other skeletal structures as well.

Static Palpation of the Head

The only joint you're checking here is the TMJ (temporomandibular joint), which, for our purposes, is the only moveable joint in the head. It is important to check the TMJ before you palpate the neck, because a misaligned jaw often indicates an atlas subluxation on the side of the deviated TMJ.

Stand directly in front of your horse. Determine if the mandible (bottom jaw) is off to one side by looking at the chin (*mentum*). If so, feel the TMJ by placing your hands in front of each ear and sliding your fingers down and towards the eyes until your feel the joint (Fig. 4-1). If necessary, have someone move the chin from side to side or open the mouth. This will enable you to feel the "hinge." If one of these sides feels larger, then your horse may have a jaw subluxation. In my experience, I have found that a right-handed horse owner will cause their horse's right TMJ to subluxate, since that person is unconsciously pulling harder on the right rein. Other signs of TMJ disorders are difficulty chewing, resisting sharp turns when pulled to the subluxated side, and frequently needing their teeth floated. (Horses develop little points on their back teeth due to irregu-

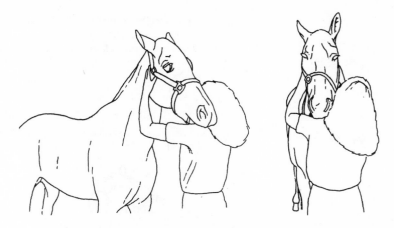

Fig. 4-1. Feeling the TMJ.

lar chewing, if their jaws aren't aligned. That's when a tooth
farrier is called in to float them, or rasp them down.) If you've
determined one side of the jaw is misaligned, coordinate your
findings by feeling the ipsilateral (same-side) atlas wing, and
see if it feels more prominent.

Static Palpation of the Neck

1. Atlas. The first two cervical vertebrae (atlas and axis) have
unique physical characteristics compared to the remaining five
neck bones. The areas of the atlas used to analyze subluxations
include the posterior (dorsal) arch and each atlas wing. Since
there are muscles covering each side of the arch, you're really
feeling for the "high-muscled" side, meaning the muscles will
feel higher and harder on that side (Fig. 4-2). If one side of the
arch feels higher, it means the overlaying muscles on that side

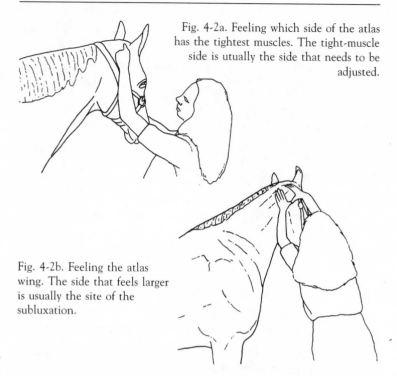

Fig. 4-2a. Feeling which side of the atlas has the tightest muscles. The tight-muscle side is utually the side that needs to be adjusted.

Fig. 4-2b. Feeling the atlas wing. The side that feels larger is usually the site of the subluxation.

have spasmed, pulling that side of the arch up which makes it "fixed" on that side. You can accentuate this high bump by slightly bending the horse's head down, further exposing the high bump. (If you ever had a wrist ganglion—a small, round growth on the back of your hand—you would notice that when you bent or flexed your wrist, the ganglion would appear bigger. This is how to imagine the posterior arch during palpation.)

Feeling for the high posterior arch may be easy for some, but is rather subjective for others. A more objective test for an atlas subluxation would be to feel the space between the atlas wing and the mandible (Fig. 4-3). For this procedure, stand in front of your horse and fit two fingers into each space. For obvious misalignments, there will be no question which space feels more snug. That side is the side of the fixation or subluxation. Simply stated, that side of the atlas wing has moved closer to the base of the skull (*occiput*), creating a narrowed space between the head and the atlas. Most equine chiropractors would agree that the atlas wings are the most easily palpated spinal prominences. Right below and to each side of the skull, the wings feel like large, chunky "skipping" stones. However, they don't quite stick out as much as Frankenstein's neck bolts, the atlas wings being a little higher.

2. Axis (Feeling the axis spinous). Two parts of the axis (second cervical) can be palpated; the tip of the spinous (spine) and the body (see Fig. 3-8). The axis spinous can be felt about

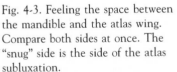
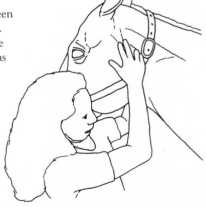

Fig. 4-3. Feeling the space between the mandible and the atlas wing. Compare both sides at once. The "snug" side is the side of the atlas subluxation.

six inches below the poll (see Fig. 3-1a). It feels like a shallow, bony ridge. Even though the axis has a long, blade-like spinous, only a few millimeters of it can be palpated. The few millimeters that can be felt with your fingers forms a little shelf emanating from the surface. For adjusting purposes, this shelf can be contacted by your *pisiform*, which is a small bone on the heel of your hand (Fig. 4-4). You can tell if the spinous is off to one side (off-center) if you can feel a tighter muscle on one side. For example, if you feel a higher and tighter muscle on the right side of the axis spinous, that means the spinous has misaligned to the right. This test isn't always accurate because sometimes the horse's spinous has natural imperfections and might have more bone material on one side, making it feel off-center. Note: A spinous that feels off-center and pointing more to one side is called a *lateral* spinous. In other words, the tip of

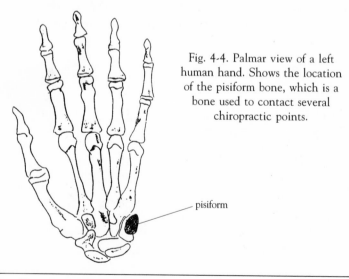

Fig. 4-4. Palmar view of a left human hand. Shows the location of the pisiform bone, which is a bone used to contact several chiropractic points.

pisiform

the spinous is pointing more to the left (left lateral) or right (right lateral). The adjustment, as you'll see in Chapter 10, is delivering a thrust or impulse in the opposite direction of spinous laterality.

The other part of the axis that can be felt is the body (see Fig. 3-7). The cervical bodies are located more towards the ventral side of the neck (throat) than towards the dorsal (mane) side. The axis body can be felt by first feeling the atlas wing and sliding your fingers down and under until you come to the first thing that feels like bone. That first thing would be the transverse process. Feel the transverse process on both sides and determine which one feels bigger. The more prominent side is the side of the axis body misalignment.

3. The rest of the neck bones. All of the other cervicals (C3 through C7) are palpated pretty much the same way as the axis body. Remember, the only cervical spinous that can be felt is the spine belonging to the axis. The remaining cervical spines are too small and too deeply embedded in the heavy neck musculature to be felt.

Static Palpation of the Mid-Back

When you look at the lateral view of a horse's skeleton, you might think the bone at the base of the neck with an elongated spinous process might be the 7th cervical. It's not! That bone is the first thoracic, or dorsal (see Fig. 3-2). Thus, the first thoracic spinous process is not easily palpated, except in emaciated animals. However, if you palpate deeply enough, you can feel the body of the first thoracic, much the same as you can feel the last cervical. For the most part, the only bony projections you can feel in the mid-back (thoracic/dorsal) vertebrae are the spinous processes. For palpation purposes, the palpation of the thoracic spine is broken down into two sections: the withers, and the rest (just like Gilligan's Island!).

The withers is the section of the dorsal spine that spans from about the top of the shoulders (T2) to the seventh dorsal. The difference in palpation between the withers and the rest of the dorsals is that you can feel more of the spinous processes in the withers—not just the tops, but a portion of the spinous sides. It is at the sides of the spines that laterality is determined. Feel the sides of the spines the best you can and ask yourself which side feels "bumpier." The bumpier side is the side to which the spinous has deviated. Determining the direction (laterality) of the dorsal spines gets a little trickier as you palpate down from the end of the withers. When you reach the 8th dorsal, the spines almost become flush with the horse's body and don't stick out as much. To determine which way the spinouses have subluxated or shifted, you have to feel the *paravertebral line*, which is a fancy way of saying the line of muscles flanking or bordering the spines (Fig. 4-5). Since you cannot feel the dorsal transverse processes, you have to rely on how the muscles feel next to each spinous. Compare the muscle texture on each side of the dorsal spinouses. Ask yourself which side feels tighter or higher. The higher side is the side of spinous deviation or spinous laterality (Fig. 4-6). **Important:** You will often notice the horse flinch with pain (tensing his abdominal muscles) while you press into the hard muscle knots. This is a sign of subluxation.

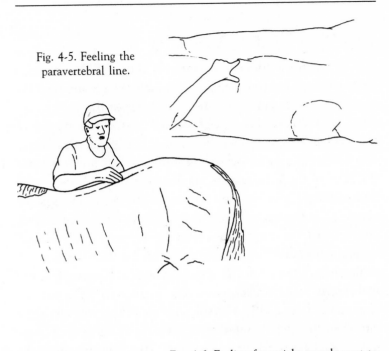

Fig. 4-5. Feeling the paravertebral line.

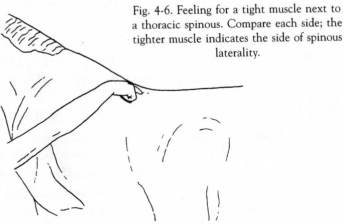

Fig. 4-6. Feeling for a tight muscle next to a thoracic spinous. Compare each side; the tighter muscle indicates the side of spinous laterality.

Static Palpation of the Lumbar Spine

Further down the thoracics, beginning with T16, you have to be on the lookout for *mammillary processes,* which are the little bony projections emanating near the sides of the spines (see Fig. 3-16). While generally not palpable in the lower thoracics, the mammillaries are palpable near the sides of the lumbar spines (the lumbar paravertebral line). As you firmly palpate the sides of the lumbars, the mammillaries feel a little harder than ordinary muscle knots. Note: When reviewing lumbar anatomy, note that you feel the mammillary processes of a vertebra first, before you reach its spinous process. So if you feel a high mammillary on the right side of the third lumbar, for example, the third lumbar spinous will be felt about half an inch down (caudal) from its own mammillary(s). The side of the high mammillary is the side *opposite* of spinous laterality. However, the high mammillary itself can be used as an adjusting contact point. By "pushing down" the high mammillary, your are essentially adjusting the lateral spinous. For example, if the mammillary is high on the right, the spinous will point to the left. Additionally, the tops of the lumbar spines feel similar to the dorsal spines (the dorsals below the withers, that is).

Static Palpation of the Sacrum

The sacrum contains a joint (the *sacroiliac* or SI joint) which connects the pelvis with the spine. The SI joint itself cannot be palpated, but four of the five fused *sacral tubercles* can be felt below the top of the hip (PSIS). The first sacral tubercle is often not palpable because it is directly beneath and between the two PSIS's. When felt with one stroke down the sacrum, the tubercles feel like speed bumps. The higher feeling side of the sacrum is the side you would adjust.

The most important part of the sacrum that can be palpated is the *sacral apex*. Chapter 13 describes one of the most important chiropractic techniques, the *Ligament Push* (a.k.a. Logan Basic Technique). The sacral apex can be felt by lifting up your horse's tail and touching a point about an inch and a half directly above, or at "12:00" to, the anus (Fig. 4-7). The Ligament Push involves contacting the *sacrotuberous ligament* from each side of the sacral apex (see Chapter 3). By some professional standards, the Ligament Push is the method of choice since it is the easiest to perform and does the most all at once.

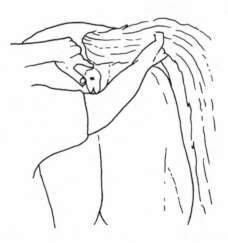

Fig. 4-7. The sacral apex can be felt at "12:00" to the anus.

Static Palpation of the Tail

Simply feel for hard muscle knots and knobby joints. The tail can best be evaluated during motion palpation.

Static Palpation of the Hips

There are two areas of the hips or pelvis that are contacted for adjusting purposes: the PSIS's or tops of the hips, and the ASIS's or sides of the hips. Each of these areas has a right and a left contact point, thus making four actual points. All of these are described in Chapter 3.

The tops of the hips, which are sometimes referred to as *tubers*, can be felt by starting at some point on the lumbar spine and running your fingers down in the direction of the tail until you come to a summit. This one little "hill" contains both tubers within a circumference about the size of a large silver dollar (the ones that predated the small Susan B. Anthony coins). Between these tubers is a split, separating them. This split is palpated as a thin crevice, underneath which lies the first sacral tubercle. The PSIS's are the contact points for most hip adjustments. When your horse is standing square on all fours, palpate these summits and determine which one feels higher. The higher tuber is most likely the side of the fixed, painful, or subluxated hip (sacroiliac joint) because the horse is trying to take pressure off that side by raising the painful leg off the ground.

The sides of the hips, which are referred to as the *point of the hips*, are called the ASIS's or *tuber coxae* (see Fig. 3-21). By simply looking at your horse's side, you can see these points sticking out. Even on a big, fleshy draft horse, the point of the hips are prominent. You can only feel one of these points at a time since they are the whole width of the horse apart. Feel one side first, then the other, and determine which side sticks out more. Feel the top of the loins on each side and stroke your way down towards the tail until you feel the ASIS. The more prominent side reflects the horse's attempt to girder a painful hip joint (*acetabular joint*) or a fixed sacroiliac joint.

Static Palpation of the Scapulas (Shoulders)

The scapulas are the horse's diaries. By looking and feeling them, you can tell where they've been. For example, a low, droopy left shoulder is the mark of a riding horse, since riding horses are mounted from their left, which causes the scapula to drop. A low shoulder is also indicative of a shoulder injury, such as a fall or a blow to the area, resulting in a condition known as *sweeney* (see Appendix A). In this condition, the nerve supply to the scapula (*suprascapular nerve*) is damaged, which weakens the surrounding muscles, thus causing the shoulder to drop. To the contrary, a high shoulder can indicate an overworked horse who consistently pulls a lopsided load. But more often than that, the high shoulder is compensating for the weaker, low shoulder, which explains why the high shoulder feels more muscular.

On a well conformed horse, the scapulas are not always visible, but they can be easily palpated by starting a point at the low cervicals (neck) and running your fingers across the shoulders (Fig. 4-8). When you reach the area above the humerus, you'll feel an isolated, hard, semi-vertical ridge. This

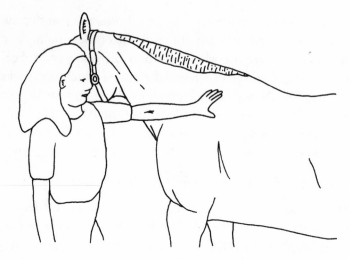

Fig. 4-8. Scanning for the scapula (shoulder blade).

long ridge is the *spine* of the scapula. Once you've located this anatomical landmark, firmly feel the outline of the scapula above, below, and to the sides of the bone. Note: Don't confuse the scapular spine with the nearby ribs, of which you can feel several at once.

Static Palpation of the Knee (Carpus)

The horse's carpus is really the physiological equivalent of our wrist, but in the horse it is called the knee. There aren't many chiropractic methods for the knee; treating knee conditions falls under veterinary domain. However, a swollen knee joint(s) can alter your gait analysis. Therefore, feel the knee with both hands and determine if one or both knees feel swollen or warm. If so, this may be the cause of lameness.

Static Palpation of the Stifle (True Knee)

This may seem elementary, but when you view a horse from the side, you might think the true knee or stifle should be found a lot lower than where it is. It is felt way above the "knee-looking" hock, upwards towards the abdomen!

The bone you want to feel here is the *patella*, or kneecap, a large sesamoid bone articulating with the lower (distal) end of the femur (thigh bone). It feels like an irregular ball. The stifle itself is the joint between the femur and tibia. But upon static palpation, determine which kneecap feels higher. An upward fixation of the patella over the end of the femur can prevent flexion of the affected hindlimb, causing the stifle and hock to "lock." This, however, is usually obvious with a quick visual inspection.

Static Palpation of the Ribs

A high-feeling rib can signal breathing problems. During the course of a strenuous race, a horse can subluxate a rib by overexpanding his rib cage. Consequently, this high rib can subluxate its vertebral attachment in the thoracic (mid-back) spine. To find the potentially subluxated mid-back bone, trace the high rib up towards the spine until you lose your tracing (about four inches from the vertebral attachment), then approximate the curve of the rib between the lost tracing point and the affected thoracic spinous (Fig. 4-9). In other words, do your best to imitate the outline of the rib curve up towards the spine. This takes practice, but is an invaluable skill once mastered.

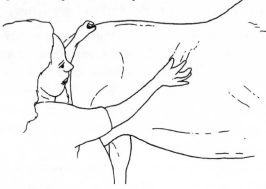

Fig. 4-9. Tracing the ribs up toward the spine.

MOTION PALPATION

Restricted joint motion is the primary sign of a subluxation. During motion palpation, you are not feeling the horse's joints while he's walking or trotting, rather, you are testing the joints in the standing horse, with and without his assistance. Watching the horse in motion is not the same as motion palpation. During motion palpation, you are skillfully feeling for areas of *hypomobility*—fixed joints that should possess fluid, effortless motion, but don't, often due to spastic muscles or physical changes in the joint from arthritis or injuries. Watching the horse in motion is part of the gait analysis (see Chapter 5).

Motion Palpation of the Neck

Motioning out and testing the neck for fixed joints is a three-step procedure. The first step is to test the *atlanto-occipital* joint, which is the joint between the base of the skull (occiput) and the first neck (cervical) bone, or atlas. The motion tested here is *extension* (chin up, head back) and *flexion* (chin down towards the chest). You might recall from Chapter 3 that the joint between the atlas and occiput is referred to as the Yes joint, since it creates the up-and-down movement of the head. A dog, unlike a horse, has quite a lot of head and neck extension and will have its nose pointing directly at the ceiling at the zenith of extension. A horse has about 65 percent as much head/neck extension as a dog.

In order to test the Yes joint, face your horse by standing directly in front of him and firmly grasp both halters (Fig. 4-10). Start with your horse's head in a neutral position. Then,

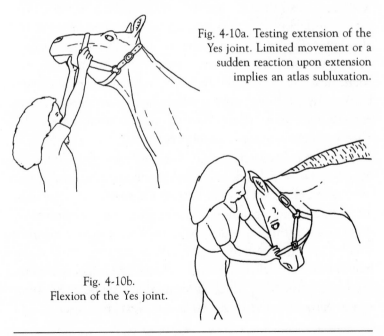

Fig. 4-10a. Testing extension of the Yes joint. Limited movement or a sudden reaction upon extension implies an atlas subluxation.

Fig. 4-10b.
Flexion of the Yes joint.

with a deliberate and even motion, guide the head up until it stops. You must proceed rather quickly, otherwise you'll give your horse a chance to resist. If your horse shows reluctance to extend his neck, check each side separately. Start again with the head in a neutral position, and grasp both halters. Proceed to lift your horse's head up as before, but halfway through, veer his head to the right and continue to lift up. Repeat for the left side. The side which appears "heavier" to lift up means the horse is resisting; the atlas is fixed on that heavier side.

After testing the Yes joint, it is time to test the No joint. This tests the *atlanto-axial* joint, which is the rotational joint between the first and second neck bones and allows the head to rotate. Head rotation is simply this: Think of a clock face. As you're facing your standing horse, note that his nose (or chin) points straight down to the "6". Left head rotation would be to move his nose up counterclockwise, toward the "5". Right head rotation would be to move his nose up clockwise, toward the "7". Restricted rotation here signifies a problem with the No joint. The axis or the second neck bone is the bone you're testing for a troubled No joint.

Once you know there's a problem with rotation, you now must find out which side of the axis is subluxated, causing the trouble. For this, you have to *laterally flex* each side of the axis. To picture lateral flexion, try touching your ear to your shoulder without lifting up your shoulder. To test lateral flexion of your horse's axis, stand to one side of him, say the left; grasp the halter with your left hand, and with your right palm contact the body of the axis, which is located directly below and beneath the atlas wing (Figs. 4-11a–c). Next, pull your horse's

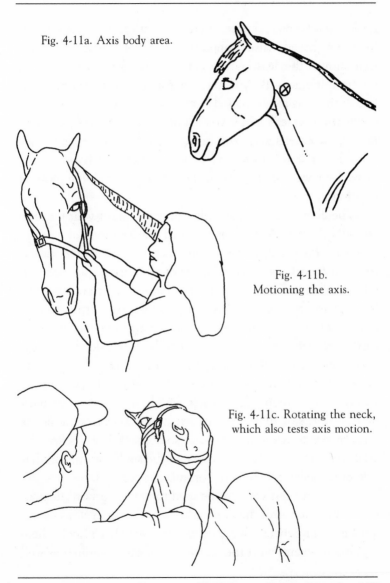

Fig. 4-11a. Axis body area.

Fig. 4-11b.
Motioning the axis.

Fig. 4-11c. Rotating the neck,
which also tests axis motion.

neck towards you and note where the motion stops. Repeat this for the right side (using opposite hands, of course). The side that moves the least is the side of the axis subluxation or fixation. Incidentally, you may test the remaining cervical vertebrae this way for decreased lateral flexion. As you test further down the cervical spine, you'll notice your horse's neck can bend quite extensively, with his nose reaching as far back as his side (flank) or at least to his shoulder. A horse with a sore neck or back may resist the lateral flexion test by moving away or backing up.

The above example describes how you assist your horse to laterally flex his neck. This is called *passive* range of motion. One clever and easy method to test cervical range of motion is to use a food bribe, such as a carrot, to entice your horse to move his neck. This is called *active* range of motion, since the horse is an actor or active part in the test. As in the example above, stand to the side of your horse and wave the aromatic carrot under his nose for a few seconds. Next, slowly pull the carrot away towards yourself, thus guiding your horse's nose until he reaches his side or shoulder (Fig. 4-12). Repeat for the opposite side, then ask yourself which side had more neck motion. The side that displayed *less* lateral flexion is the side of a cervical subluxation, that is, of some neck bone below the atlas. Now that you know the side of the subluxation, feel that side of the neck for the more prominent cervical.

The carrot test can also be used to detect forward flexion, by waving the carrot under your horse's nose then slowly guiding his head between his forelegs (Fig. 4-13). Difficulty here suggests problems with the atlas (part of the Yes joint) as well

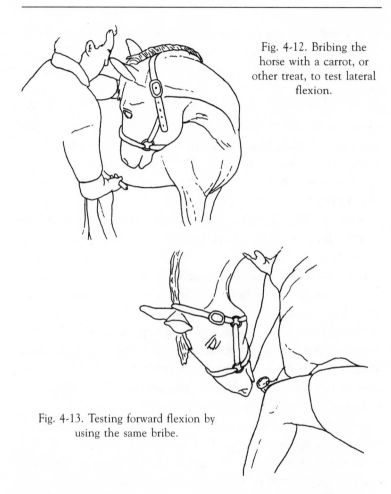

Fig. 4-12. Bribing the horse with a carrot, or other treat, to test lateral flexion.

Fig. 4-13. Testing forward flexion by using the same bribe.

as the spinouses belonging to the first or second thoracic (mid-back) bone. The reason the first or second thoracic would be involved is because that is where the *nuchal* ligament attaches. If you recall, the nuchal ligament acts as sort of an extension bridge between the head and the upper mid-back. A subluxation of the first or second thoracic can cause an irregular pull on this ligament, affecting neck flexion.

Motion Palpation of the Mid-Back Bones (Thoracics)

With the exception of the first thoracic spinous (which is difficult, if not impossible, to palpate), the upper thoracics, or withers area, may be motioned out by grasping the long tips of each spinous process up to about the 7th thoracic (the end of the withers). After the 7th thoracic, the spinouses become shorter and flush with the body, so they can't be grasped. So, to test the motion of the 2nd through 7th thoracics, stand to the side of your horse and test each spinous separately by pulling them toward you, one at a time (Figs. 4-14a–b). They don't exactly wiggle like a loose tooth, but you will notice which one(s) fights the pulling more. If, for example, you're standing at the left side of your horse, and you're pulling a spinous from right to left which shows resistance, you'll know that particular spinous is fixed on the right and will ultimately have to be adjusted by standing on the right side and pushing that spinous from right to left (see Chapter 11).

To motion-palpate the lower thoracics (just below the shoulders), stand to the side of your horse with the base of your hand to the side of the spinouses and your other hand grasping the base of the tail (Fig. 4-15). Next, pull the base of the tail towards yourself as you motion (laterally push) each spinous. You should notice an easy give to the spine. Repeat this procedure on the other side. The areas of the spine that gives or bends the least is the side of the fixation and/or subluxation.

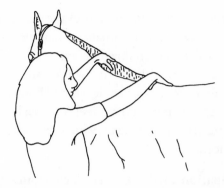

Fig. 4-14a. Scanning the upper thoracics for tight muscles next to the spine.

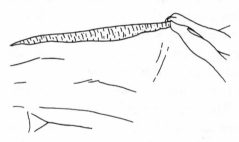

Fig. 4-14b. Motioning the upper thoracics by pulling them towards you.

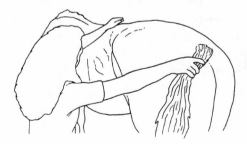

Fig. 4-15. Motioning the mid- to lower thoracics by grasping the base of the tail, using it as an anchor.

Another way to test the motion of the mid- to lower thoracics is to stand on a couple of bales of hay, elevating yourself above your horse, and push down on each spinous, testing the "springs." Healthy spinal ligaments will create a cushiony but firm environment for the vertebrae which allows for flexibility. As you push each spinous down, feel for "dead" spots, or the spinal segments that flex the least, which are usually the sites of the subluxations.

Motion Palpation of the Lower Back Bones (Lumbars)

The last rib indicates the area of the last thoracic; just below that is the beginning of the low back, or lumbars. The lumbars are motioned out exactly the same way as the mid- and lower thoracics, with the addition of two other methods.

The first of these additional methods is to firmly stroke down your horse's lumbar spine until you reach the sacrum (Fig. 4-16). The horse's natural response to this is to *ventroflex* or hollow out his lower back. Once you get this response, test

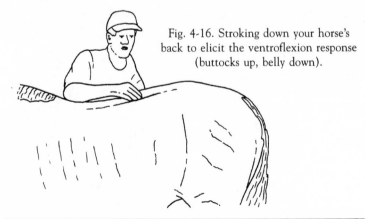

Fig. 4-16. Stroking down your horse's back to elicit the ventroflexion response (buttocks up, belly down).

each side by firmly stroking each area individually. A quicker, more dramatic response can be a sign of pain. This, however, isn't always the case. A horse exhibiting no ventroflexion in response to the firm stroking may have tighter muscles there and could be in too much spasm to respond. Therefore, you'll have to look for other responses, such as kicking, whining, or pulling away.

The second of these two methods is to firmly stroke the *croup* (the area between the hips and the point of the buttocks) with a semi-blunt object, like a ballpoint pen with its pointy cover on (Fig. 4-17). The response should be *dorsiflexion*, or arching of the *thoracolumbar* region. If you don't get this response, your horse may have tight mid- and lower back muscles. Similarly, stroking the pen (or your fingertips) underneath your horse (in his abdominal area) will also cause your horse to arch his back; in some cases, sustaining this irritation and retaining this arch for a minute or two can actually help relieve back

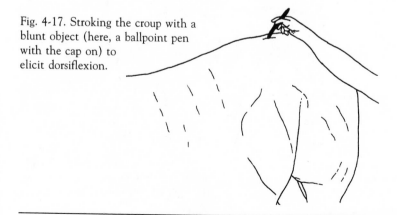

Fig. 4-17. Stroking the croup with a blunt object (here, a ballpoint pen with the cap on) to elicit dorsiflexion.

pain. Lastly, stroking the pen on the side of the back (the lateral thoracic or lumbar area) will normally cause your horse's spine to move (flex) away from the irritation.

Motion Palpation of the Hips

Motioning the hips is really a test for the sacroiliac (SI) joint. To test for aberrant hip motion, elevate yourself over your horse by standing on a couple of bales of hay. Next, feel the PSIS's, which as you'll recall are the two little hills felt below the last lumbar (Fig. 4-18). Push down on each of these bumps and notice which one "gives" the least. That one would be the fixed SI joint. An even better motion test is to see which hind leg extends back the least (Fig. 4-19). That one would be the side of the fixed SI joint. **Warning: Grasping and extending**

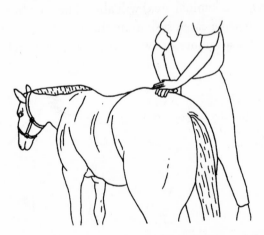

Fig. 4-18. Motioning the sacroiliac joint (from atop some bales of hay) by pushing down on the top of the hips (PSIS's). The hip that gives the least is the side of the subluxated SI joint.

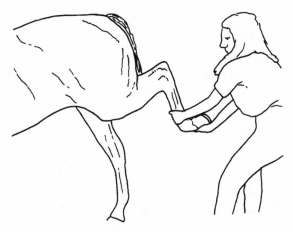

Fig. 4-19. Testing the sacroiliac joint by extending the hind legs backward, one at a time (with extreme caution!). The leg that extends the least is the side of the sacroiliac subluxation.

the hind legs can be dangerous. Proceed with caution or get someone else to do it (for example, someone who owes you money).

Motion Palpation of the Sacrum

Again, you are testing the SI joint. To test the SI joint by using the sacrum, it's best to remain standing and elevated next to your horse. With one hand, push the end of the sacrum down, while your other hand feels both PSIS's (Fig. 4-20). To test the right SI joint, push the right end of the sacrum down and feel if the right PSIS "pokes" into your hand. Repeat for the left SI joint. The PSIS that springs up the least, or not at all, is the side of the fixed SI joint.

Motion Palpation of the Tail

With the tail in a drooped and relaxed position, you should be able to effortlessly lift it up while grasping it at the center (Fig. 4-21). A tail that feels rigid, like fiberglass, is a sign of low-back pain.

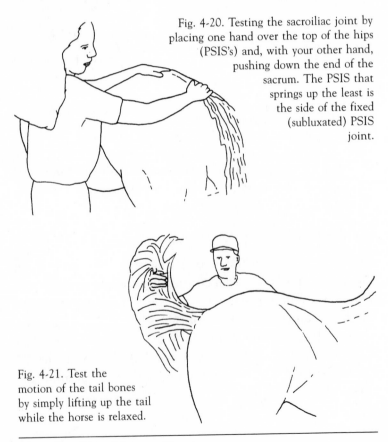

Fig. 4-20. Testing the sacroiliac joint by placing one hand over the top of the hips (PSIS's) and, with your other hand, pushing down the end of the sacrum. The PSIS that springs up the least is the side of the fixed (subluxated) PSIS joint.

Fig. 4-21. Test the motion of the tail bones by simply lifting up the tail while the horse is relaxed.

Motion Palpation of the Shoulders (Scapulas)

The scapulas are sites for muscle attachments and don't form true shoulder joints since the horse has no clavicles (collar-bones). Therefore, when testing for scapular motion, you are actually testing their range of motion within their own muscu-lature. Since they can only be restricted by tight muscles, you have to determine how far they can "swim." There are two motion tests for the scapulas. The first test (Figs. 4-22a–b) is to stand to the side of your horse next to a front leg, bend his knee

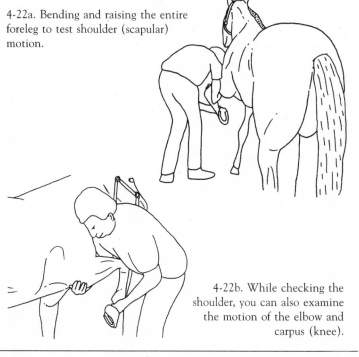

4-22a. Bending and raising the entire foreleg to test shoulder (scapular) motion.

4-22b. While checking the shoulder, you can also examine the motion of the elbow and carpus (knee).

(carpus), and raise up the entire limb. That front leg's scapula should rise so the top of it is level with the withers. Test the other side and compare. The scapula that doesn't rise as high is the side of increased muscle tightness, and needs to be adjusted. The second scapular motion test (Figs. 4-23a–b) is to grasp the lower front leg and move forward until you're in front of the horse. This stretching exercise will lower the scapula down on the rib cage. Again, test the other side and compare. The scapula that lowered the least is the side of the restriction.

Motion Palpation of the Knees

I am referring here to the front knees, or the carpus (our wrist equivalent). While standing to the side of your horse, raise the cannon and flex the knee (Figs. 4-24a–b). Compare each side.

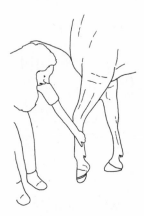

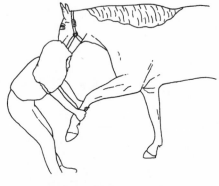

Fig. 4-23a. Bending the knee to raise the foreleg.

Fig. 4-23b. Stretching the foreleg forward to lower the scapula down on the rib cage. The sacpula that lowers the least is the side of the shoulder restriction.

The knee that flexes (bends) the least is either swollen and/or needs to be adjusted.

The "true knee," or stifle, can be examined for tenderness by cupping your hand around the patella, or kneecap (Fig. 4-25), as described in Chapter 3.

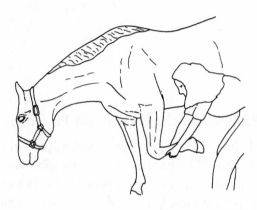

Fig. 4-24a. You can test knee motion by simply lifting up on the cannon.

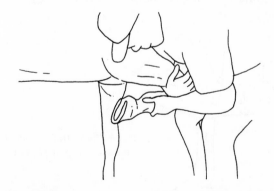

Fig. 4-24b. Some practitioners flex the knee all the way to test motion.

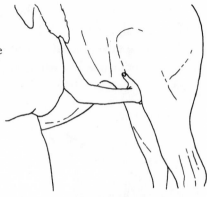

Fig. 4-25. Examining the stifle (true knee).

Motion Palpation of the Fetlock and Pastern Joints

The fetlock joint is located between the long pastern bone and the cannon bone. The pastern joint is the joint between the short pastern bone and the long pastern bone. Both the front and hind legs have these bones and joints. Normal movement of these areas are vital for fluid walking and trotting. Motion out each joint and compare both sides (Fig. 4-26).

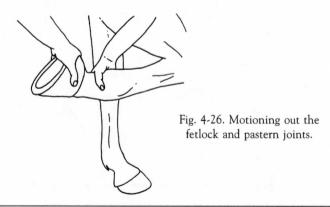

Fig. 4-26. Motioning out the fetlock and pastern joints.

Motion Palpation of the Hock

While the hock joint does display some motion, it is difficult to motion out. Therefore, I suggest that you simply feel the hock joint and determine if one side is more swollen than the other. If so, the more swollen side would express less motion.

Motion Palpation of the TMJ (Jaw)

A fixed temporomandibular joint can cause neck subluxations, particularly of the atlas. To test the TMJ, situate yourself in front of your horse and grasp the lower part of the mandible, or lower jaw bone (Fig. 4-27). Gently push the mandible up towards the ears until you feel the jaw muscles relaxing (about 30 seconds). Then, rock the jaw from side to side and note which side rocks more. The side that rocks the least is the side of the fixed or subluxated TMJ. It is also the side of the subluxated atlas.

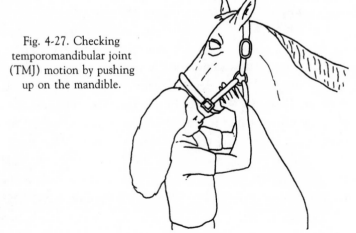

Fig. 4-27. Checking temporomandibular joint (TMJ) motion by pushing up on the mandible.

CHAPTER 5

EQUINE CHIROPRACTIC EXAMINATION

This chapter might be entitled, "How do you know when your horse needs to be adjusted?" This is the question most commonly asked by the person sitting next to me on a plane. The only people who never ask it are other chiropractors. They already know. A horse, like any other mammal, needs to be adjusted when normal joint function/movement has been restricted by the natural barriers, namely the muscles and ligaments surrounding the joints.

Funk & Wagnall's Standard College Dictionary defines *examine* as "to inspect or scrutinize with care," as well as "to subject (a person, organ, etc.) to medical scrutiny, and testing." I generally don't like to use the term *medical* to describe a chiropractic procedure. While not entirely inaccurate, the term implies an allopathic process—treating symptoms, not causes. The goal of the chiropractic examination is not to diagnose and name specific diseases, but to determine and evaluate if the patient is structurally sound. Where does the Tin Man need oil?

The phrase I like to use when discerning abnormal function of the joint being tested is *aberrant motion.* Did the joint stray from its normal function? Does it move like it should? If not, why? These are the questions you want to ask yourself while performing the equine chiropractic examination. A good household example that depicts aberrant motion is when you pull out a desk drawer that sticks and stops on the way out, but opens nonetheless. Sure, you can live with this drawer the way it is. But wouldn't it be nice if that drawer pulled out smoothly without your having to fight it each time?

This is a common example of aberrant motion, but it's not entirely accurate when discussing living tissue. The desk will become whole at once when the drawer is repaired. But when part of a living being isn't functioning properly, the whole suffers for a period after the faulty part is fixed. The body takes time to heal. It needs to recover. Finding and restoring the bad cog is only the first step in the biomechanical healing process. The *chiropractic eye* is focused on finding and removing the subluxation. Once normalcy has returned to the subluxated joint, the rest of the body can "un-compensate" and return to normal as well.

To be sure, a vertebral subluxation isn't the only cause of fixed and less vital joints. In humans, arthritis is the primary reason why people feel stiff and sluggish—older people especially. When I first started practicing, the advice from others was to establish an office in a neighborhood full of elderly people, reasoning that they need chiropractic care more since their joints hurt more. This really isn't true. After middle age, the body degenerates at a fairly predictable rate. The joints simply wear out from a lifetime of use and hurt more while attempting youthful activities. They're not supposed to move as much. Accepting who you are at any time of life, not trying to stay "young," is half the battle of staying healthy. Much of the New Age thinking that an 80-year-old man shouldn't have to slow down—"Doggone it, I'm going to go bungee jumping and you can't tell me I can't"—is society's way of telling this man he shouldn't come to grips with his own mortality. Maybe this guy should be put out to stud, like they do with horses when their racing careers end. While some senior citizens can lift weights and thrive in the process, they are the exception. The bottom line is, just be who you are.

The majority of my human practice is comprised of people in the 18 to 45 age range. They are the most active—the ones who participate in sports, climb mountains, and work out in the gym. Older people have more medical conditions than young people: heart disease, high blood pressure, and diabetes, to name a few. Chiropractors usually don't treat these conditions. Active people, like horses, are candidates for subluxations. Any movement you make is another opportunity for a muscle to splint the vertebral joint that went just a little too far in your quest to enjoy life. But here's the rub. Horses become subluxated in our quest to enjoy *them!* In the wild, horses don't spontaneously bolt 35 miles per hour for exactly one mile to try to beat another horse to a predetermined finish line just to win a prize. They also wouldn't voluntarily stand in one place for hours at a time, getting stiff in the stall. Furthermore, horses in nature don't just happen to stumble upon a rich cache of high-protein oats every day and eat it all at once. We force our will on these gentle creatures in several ways; making them carry saddles, chomping on bits, kicking them with spurs, restricting them with harnesses—just to name a few. To us, these are the tools of a trade. To them, they're S&M devices.

Let's not get into a heady discussion on man's inhumanity to animals. After all, we don't breed animals just so they can enjoy themselves. Most people would argue that these animals wouldn't be here at all if we didn't want them for our own use. As long as that's the case, and it is, we must deal with the hand we have dealt them. Just as the choke collar is detrimental to a dog's neck, the implements we compel the horse to wear, which we call *tack*, can be equally harmful and must be considered in the equine examination.

There are six parts to a chiropractic examination: *case history, posture analysis, gait analysis, static palpation, motion palpation,* and *muscle palpation.* When evaluating your horse for subluxations, all of these must be considered, in the order given. Let's explore each part.

1. CASE HISTORY

Most clinicians will tell you the case history is the single most important part of any health care examination. You must first know where the patient's been before you know where he's going. Points to ponder while studying the horse's history include age, sex, breed, occupation, medical history (medications and past or present lameness), and current complaint. Knowing a little about the previous owner(s), if there was one, would also be beneficial.

The age of the horse has a great deal to do with your evaluation. From a chiropractic standpoint, older horses move slower and their joints are stiffer. This is, in part, due to arthritis (joint inflammation). Additionally, older horses tend to lose muscle tone from lack of exercise. A horse lacking proper muscle tone responds less favorably to chiropractic care compared to a horse who's allowed to exercise. Weak muscles and ligaments cannot adequately support a rigid back. Horses, at any age, should be regularly exercised in accordance with their abilities. An older horse showing his age may exhibit protruding withers, drooping shoulders, or a swayed back. Many of these characteristics could be prevented or lessened with regular exercise. Young horses and foals should be checked for subluxations due to possible birth trauma. This is particularly important before the commencement of any training regiment.

The sex of the horse should be taken into consideration. A mare with cystic ovaries, for example, may show signs of back pain. Also, during her last few months of gestation, the ligaments are more relaxed in the mare, and therefore less adjusting force is required. The male horse, or stallion, will have trouble mounting the mare if he has back pain.

Knowledge of the horse's breed and body type is a vital component of the case history. *Limitations* is the buzzword here. Abilities differ with body type. Just as a squat-bodied, short-legged Bulldog cannot run as fast as a streamlined, wispy Greyhound—a lumbering, cold-blooded, heavy-footed Clydesdale cannot compete on the racetrack with a chiseled, hot-blooded Thoroughbred. Also, some breeds are predisposed for certain conditions, albeit rare. For example, some Arabians may be afflicted with a congenital malformation of the *atlanto-occipital* joint, in which the base of the skull (occiput) is fused with the first neck bone (the atlas), often resulting in spinal cord compression and an irregular gait. A more common cervical condition, seen mostly in Thoroughbreds, is *wobbler syndrome*. This, too, creates an irregular gait and spinal cord compression.

The horse's occupation is another piece of the case history puzzle. A *jumper* who leaps over hurdles, for example, may dislocate his sacroiliac joint and exhibit a "bump" over his hip (Fig. 5-1). A horse working at a riding stable who's forced to carry a different size person every day, will have more back problems and left shoulder strains (because the riders mount the horse from his left side).

While scrutinizing the horse's body, you must consider his past medical history which includes prior lameness, medications, boarding environment, and psychological makeup. The latter has more to do with how well he was treated or mistreated by his previous owners. Some types of lameness can have a long-term effect on the horse's health and performance if not properly treated. *Navicular disease*, for instance, is a common forelimb lameness often afflicting the Quarter horse and Thoroughbred, especially geldings (castrated male horses). With

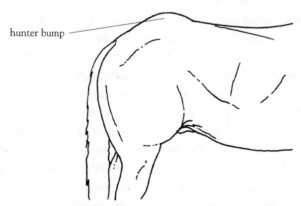

hunter bump

Fig. 5-1. Hunter bump: a sacroiliac luxation or dislocation common among hunter-jumper horses.

this disease, or lameness, there is damage to the *navicular* bone (a small bone near the foot), which could be caused by prolonged working on hard surfaces, improper trimming of the feet, or *ischemic necrosis* (blood deficiency causing tissue death). Now the diagnostic pattern starts to emerge; knowing that past or present lameness alters the gait will allow you to be more critical and forgiving during your analysis and treatment.

Medications such as *phenylbutazone* ("bute"), which is a nonsteroidal anti-inflammatory drug (NSAID), and pain killers will mask musculoskeletal symptoms, thus altering your evaluation and treatment. When you're "under the influence," you don't even know when you're experiencing pain. I often think about this when I leave the dentist's office with my tongue still numb from Novocaine. Crunching into your tongue seems perfectly natural when you first leave the office. "Hey, I can handle that." But your bravery turns to horror later on that night when you discover the wounds you've inflicted on yourself.

Generally, if the horse is on medication, he is under veterinary care, unless the owner himself is administering drugs. It is not unusual for the owner or trainer to act as a secondary vet and assume the lion's share of health care responsibilities. In the time I've spent in stables, I've seen trainers drain abscesses, treat skin ulcers, even give injections—sometimes right before a race! However, I rarely see the owners or trainers perform dental work (floating). When a horse grinds his food by moving his jaws from side to side, little enamel points can develop on the upper and lower rows of teeth. These sharp points can cause the horse much discomfort, such as tongue and cheek abrasions, thus the horse will eat less due to the pain. Teeth problems also cause the jaw to become misaligned, which in turn causes the neck muscles to spasm. A competent trainer will call in a vet or a professional tooth farrier to do the dental work.

The same holds true for foot problems. The number one cause of lameness not due to injury or disease is improper shoeing and foot care. A good blacksmith is worth his weight in gold. He is your horse mechanic, and you need to hire the best one available. After all, you wouldn't put just any tire on a valuable sports car. Just as your car tires need to be rotated and checked for thin treads, your horse's feet and hoofs need to be regularly maintained—and not by a hacker. I don't know how many times I've seen an otherwise sound horse lose the race due to a shoe nail too close to the *frog*, the sensitive underside of the hoof.

All of this is a prelude to why the horse needs your help in the first place—his present condition. Why is he walking funny? Is it due to an improperly fitting saddle? Is his stall too confining and doesn't allow enough room to stretch out? Does he have a medical or a chiropractic condition? This is probably the most important question. Even though most horse lameness conditions are due to leg and foot problems, you still have to watch the horse in motion—taking the lameness into consideration. Chiropractic is about restoring normal motion to the body, especially the joints, not forming a medical diagnosis. Veterinarians do that. After you know the horse's chief complaint or condition, you have to watch him in motion. In other words, analyze his gait and posture. How solid is his foundation?

2. POSTURE ANALYSIS

The most apropos word to describe how the standing and re-laxed horse should look is *conformation*. While standing on all fours, the horse should appear symmetrical, like a solid table that doesn't need cardboard placed under the legs so it won't wobble. Let's look at some of the asymmetrical signs of faulty posture and the areas of the body affected:

1. **Head:** The horse's jaw (mandible) will deviate (get off-center) to one side if he has head pain, teeth pain, or problems with the temporomandibular joint (TMJ).
2. **Neck:** A tilted head could mean neck pain.
3. **Mid-back:** If you notice the horse has a *lordosis* (sway-back), he could have thoracic (mid-back) pain, or just be getting old. Also, foreleg toes that are wearing down can also be a sign of mid-back pain.
4. **Low back:** A swayback also affects the low back. Un-usual wear of the rear leg toe(s) can also be a sign of low back pain.
5. **Hip:** While viewing the horse from behind, note if the top of one of his hips appears higher. The higher hip implies pain on that side.
6. **Stifle (the "rear leg" knee):** A perpetually raised rear leg often means stifle pain.
7. **Hock:** If one of the rear legs is pulled under, that could imply a painful hock on that side.
8. **Foreleg:** If the forelegs are pulled under, it could mean

navicular pain in the foreleg(s). This stance shows the horse trying to take pressure off the navicular bone, which is a small bone of the foot.

3. Gait Analysis

The word *gait* refers to the manner in which the horse moves, such as a walk, pace, trot, canter, and gallop. These are considered the *natural gaits*. Here is a brief description of these gaits.

1. **Walk:** The walk is a four-beat gait with an even rhythm. The sequence of the walk is as follows: left hind, left front, right hind, right front (Fig. 5-2). Sometimes a horse will rush at the walk and exhibit an impure gait called *prancing*, which is a combination of walking and trotting.

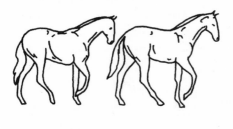

Fig. 5-2. The walk: a four-beat gait with even rhythm.

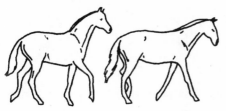

2. **Pace:** The pace is a fast two-beat lateral gait in which the two right limbs rise and land alternately with the two left limbs (Fig. 5-3). The pace is considered to be an impure gait because it breaks the natural four-beat walking gait. The pace is often associated with the Standardbred race horse.

3. **Trot:** The trot is a two-beat diagonal gait where opposite fore and hind limbs hit the ground simultaneously (Fig. 5-4). This is considered the horse's steadiest and most rhythmic gait.

4. **Canter:** The canter (lope) is a three-beat gait seen often with Western pleasure riding. The sequence of the canter is as follows: one hind limb, then the other hind limb simultaneously with its diagonal forelimb, and finally the remaining forelimb (Fig. 5-5).

5. **Gallop:** The gallop, a four-beat variation of the canter, is how the horse runs. The limbs are fully extended with the propulsion coming from the rear. The in-

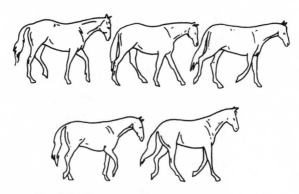

Fig. 5-3. The pace: a fast two-beat lateral gait.

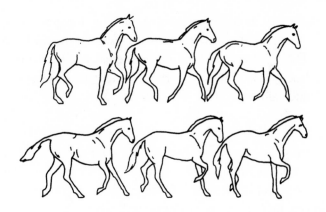

Fig. 5-4. The trot: a two-beat diagonal gait.

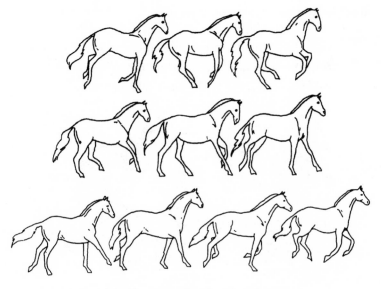

Fig. 5-5. The canter (lope): a three-beat gait.

creased impulsion or pushing along with the length of stride, the diagonal pair breaks, resulting in four beats. There is a certain "footfall" sequence, of which a right lead gallop would be: left hind, right hind, left front, and right front (Fig. 5-6).

The Abnormal Gait

Only a trained eye can analyze an abnormal gait. Every trainer I've met *has* a trained eye. Most trainers have been around several types of horses and have seen all of the gaits in action. However, most horse owners primarily know how their own horse moves. The equine chiropractor's eye should at least know when a horse is out of sequence and why. Let's briefly consider the most common reasons a horse is out of sync.

1. **The short reach:** While viewing the horse trotting from the side, note the maximum reach of each hind leg, which is really the place where the hind foot

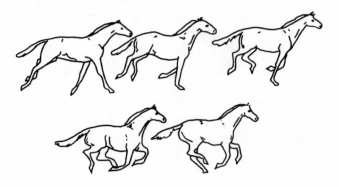

Fig. 5-6. The gallop: a four-beat variation of the canter.

touches the ground. The leg with the shorter reach is usually the side of the painful hip or sacroiliac joint.

2. **Head bobbing or nodding:** The horse's head will nod as the painful foreleg hits the ground.

3. **Hip rising or hiking:** As the painful hind leg strikes the ground, the ipsilateral (same-side) hip will come up in order to relieve pressure on that side.

4. **Inward arc of one rear leg:** Usually means low-back or hock pain.

5. **Outward arc of one rear leg:** Usually implies stifle or hip pain.

6. **Inward arc of one foreleg:** Usually implies knee pain.

7. **Outward arc of one foreleg:** Usually means shoulder or back pain.

4~5. STATIC AND MOTION PALPATION

See Chapter 4 for instructions.

Conformation

As a convenience for the reader, I've included in this section a few diagrams that depict incorrect conformation in the lower back and hindquarters (Fig. 5-7), along with foreleg and hind leg defects (Fig. 5-8a–b). As the word implies, there should be a predictable form to the horse, a form that compliments his use and the needs of his owners. Figure 3-1a (p. 30) closely resembles what a normal horse should look like.

The various defects, whether inherent or acquired, should be carefully scrutinized before buying a horse or asking him to

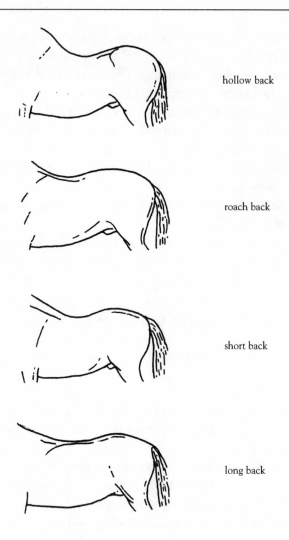

hollow back

roach back

short back

long back

Fig. 5-7. Conformation defects. Any of these defects can cause back pain and/or impaired performance.

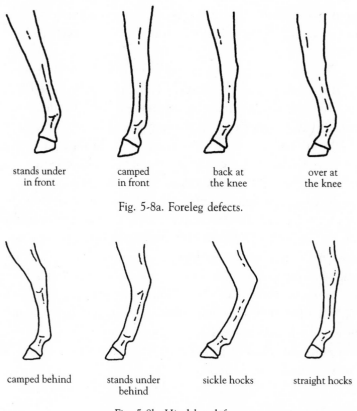

stands under
in front

camped
in front

back at
the knee

over at
the knee

Fig. 5-8a. Foreleg defects.

camped behind

stands under
behind

sickle hocks

straight hocks

Fig. 5-8b. Hind leg defects.

perform a certain task. Horses with long backs, for example, are subject to strain and inflammation. A sway or hollow back indicates ligament weakness and/or arthritis. Likewise, a horse with an arched (roach) back may be predisposed to arthritis and a faulty gait in his hind legs. This doesn't, of course, mean a badly conformed horse is useless. For example, when a horse is no longer suited for racing, he is often given another occupation such as pleasure riding which may suit his body type just fine.

The shape of the legs is important too. A horse should stand fairly square. A pigeon-toed (toe in) or splayfooted (toe out) horse will have impeded movement, which affects the whole body. A leg defect can cause sore tendons and ligaments, which can lead to muscle tension and pain. In turn, the horse has to work harder to accomplish the same tasks, causing him to fatigue quicker than a normally formed horse.

As you can imagine, conformation faults can have a significant impact on all the muscles, including the back. This is why you should seek advice not only from your horse vet but also from your farrier before you draw any examination conclusions. Find out why your horse is standing and walking abnormally. A well-trained farrier can advise you on proper leg and back conformation as well as corrective shoeing, which is paramount for a well-aligned horse. For more information on conformation and proper shoeing, I suggest you read *Shoeing Right* by David Krolick (Breakthrough, 1991).

6. MUSCLE PALPATION

With muscle palpation you're looking for a variation of skin textures with your hands and a pain response with your eyes. The horse should be standing and as relaxed as possible naturally (i.e., not under the influence of drugs). Gently feel each area of the horse's musculature, beginning with the head (TMJ) and work your way down the neck, forelegs, mid-back, sides, lower back, flank, buttocks, hips, hind legs, and tail. Feel for tight and tender muscle fibers, swelling, and skin lesions—not that you'll be treating skin lesions, but if you find one, you'll know it's not a musculoskeletal problem. Tight skin implies tight muscles. But horses' muscles are naturally tight, so you must palpate and compare both sides. Weak, flaccid muscles imply a loss of nerve supply to the muscles. Cold-feeling skin could be caused by a lack of blood supply to the muscles, in which case gentle massage may be in order.

After you've made your gentle palpation pass around the horse, you're ready to firm up your touch and test for pain. I'm not talking about digging into his body, which would cause harm, but enough pressure (between 5 to 10 lbs.) to elicit a response. Judging the response is a little tricky. Horses have a *fly swatter reflex* that can be misread as a pain signal. With a fly swatter response, you'll usually see only the skin ripple. With pain, however, the horse will quickly move away, raise up a limb, or cry out. Don't worry, he'll let you know when you've hurt him! Chiropractors refer to this procedure as *nerve tracing*. It's not that you can actually feel a nerve like a cord or a string. Rather, you look for signs that a nerve is impinged—pain being the ultimate indicator; once you know where the muscle hurts, you can trace the muscle back to its general spinal origin and adjust the subluxated vertebra.

There are some chiropractic schools that teach nerve tracing as a form of *visceral* (internal organ) diagnosis. This form of diagnosis is called the *meric system*, so named because the various tissue zones of the body are known in chiropractic terms as *meres*. This is not as confusing as it sounds. The theory is based on the fact that a spinal nerve, where it emerges at the inter-vertebral foramen (IVF; see Fig. 3-19), has branches leading to muscles (motor branches) and branches which lead to internal organs. The fact that these two nerve branches came out of the same hole in the spine, also means they were related when they left the spinal cord. Now, you can't feel the deeper nerve branches which lead to the viscera, but you *can* feel the outside of the horse and test the outer nerve branches for pain by pushing into the muscles. If the kidney was ailing, for example, its nerve "brother" on the side of the horse's back would elicit muscle pain. This theory was accidentally discovered while studying *herpes zoster* (shingles), which is a viral disease char-acterized by skin eruptions and pain along the course of the involved sensory nerves. The involved skin area's innervation was traced to the involved spinal nerve, which in turn was traced to the involved organ. The correlations proved to be much more than coincidental. This is not to say that you can diagnose an exact internal disease by using this system, but at least you can guess there's something wrong with an organ.

The above discussion of the equine chiropractic examina-tion is by no standards complete. It should simply be used as a guide—or a cursory glance, if you will—to locating potential musculoskeletal problems that may respond to chiropractic care. Remember, no animal examination is complete without a quali-fied veterinary opinion.

As always, proper documentation is a necessary compo-nent of any health care examination. Use the forms on the next two pages as an aid to your evaluation.

EXAMINATION FORM

Owner's Complaint: _____

_____

Location of Problem: _____

Duration of Problem: _____

Onset of Problem: _____

Exacerbated By (what makes it worse):

_____

_____

Remised By (what makes it better):

_____

_____

Present Medications: _____

_____

Previous Diagnostic Work (by whom):

_____

_____

Previous Medical or Chiropractic
Treatment: _____

_____

_____

Past Conditions: _____

_____

_____

_____
Date

_____
Horse's Name

_____
Owner

_____

_____
Address

_____
Phone Number

Spinal Curvatures: Normal _____
Kyphotic (arching) _____
Lordotic (swayback) _____
Scoliosis (curvature to one side):
  Right _____ Left_____
Abnormal Posture: *Where?* _____

_____
Gait Analysis: *Which leg/hip affected?*

_____
Muscular System: *Palpation/Observation*
Atrophy _____
Weakness _____
Incoordination _____
Pain/Tenderness _____
Range of Motion: *Restricted area/side:*
Cervical _____
Thoracic _____
Lumbar _____
Sacro-pelvic _____
Extremity _____
Other Findings _____

_____

_____

SPINAL EXAMINATION

_____
Horse's Name

_____
Owner

_____
Date

LEGEND:
MK=Muscle Knot
HS=Hot Spot
FJ=Fixed Joint
C=Compensation Area
P=Pain
S=Subluxation

Note: You may use none or all of the abbreviations for any vertebral area. Just write them next to the specified bone.

_____	C1	_____
_____	C2	_____
_____	C3	_____
_____	C4	_____
_____	C5	_____
LEFT _____	C6	_____ RIGHT
_____	C7	_____
_____	T1	_____
_____	T2	_____
_____	T3	_____
_____	T4	_____
_____	T5	_____
_____	T6	_____
_____	T7	_____
_____	T8	_____
_____	T9	_____
_____	T10	_____
_____	T11	_____
_____	T12	_____
_____	T13	_____
_____	T14	_____
_____	T15	_____
_____	T16	_____
_____	T17	_____
_____	T18	_____
_____	L1	_____
_____	L2	_____
_____	L3	_____
_____	L4	_____
_____	L5	_____
_____	L6	_____
_____ LEFT HIP	RIGHT HIP	_____
_____	S1	_____
_____	S2	_____
_____	S3	_____
_____	S4	_____
_____	S5	_____
_____	TAIL	_____

Chapter 6

Contraindications

Contraindications are reasons why you shouldn't use chiropractic manipulation on your horse. This refers specifically to those methods that require thrusting into a joint or the use of traction. Soft-tissue methods, such as the Ligament Push (Logan Basic Technique) or trigger-point techniques, are safe to do under most circumstances.

The primary contraindication is utilizing chiropractic methods for conditions that generally don't respond to this treatment, thus delaying the use of appropriate therapies. This is why your horse should be thoroughly checked by a veterinarian *before* administering any chiropractic procedures.

Horses, for the most part, are hardy creatures and can easily absorb the force of an adjustment as long as it is performed by hand, as opposed to with hammers or mallets. The number one reason why you would refrain from adjusting your horse is safety. Never put yourself or your horse in danger. A hysterical, or otherwise jumpy, horse should not be adjusted until that period is over. There is *never* a situation where safety overrides the need to adjust a horse.

Most contraindications are just plain common sense and apply not only to horses, but to just about any animal who can benefit from a chiropractic adjustment.

1. **Fractures.** Never adjust a bone that has an un-healed fracture, or a bone near such a fracture. A broken bone renders the whole animal unstable, and therefore too unpredictable.

2. **Recent trauma.** Any type of trauma or injury is the horse owner's nightmare. A horse should be thoroughly checked by a vet immediately following trauma, before any manual healing methods, including chiropractic, are performed.

3. **Stress.** A horse can get stressed by so many things, including confrontations with other animals, a grueling race, lack of attention, difficult training sessions, and nervous people, to name a few. If you perceive the stressful situation is temporary, allow your horse a cooling off period before adjusting him.

4. **Vascular (vein and artery) conditions (Rare).** Hardening of the arteries, strokes, and *myocardial infarctions* (heart attacks) are uncommon in horses. A more common equine vascular malady is *thrombophlebitis* of the jugular vein, a vein near the neck/throat. This condition is iatrogenic (doctor-induced) since it is caused by repeated jugular vein puncture while obtaining blood samples. The physical irritation caused by the instrument (*catheter*) inserted into the blood vessel can cause inflammation (*phlebitis*) and ultimately a blood clot (*thrombus*) in a section of the vein. This contraindication applies mainly to cervical adjusting, for the purpose of averting strokes (*cerebral vascular accidents*). However, this problem is more common with elderly

human patients than with animals. And according to some estimates, the chance of a stroke occurring during cervical manipulation of a human being is less than one in ten million adjustments.

5. **Tumors.** The possibility of causing a fracture by rendering an adjustment is increased in the cancer patient, especially if the bone itself is malignant. Albeit rare, malignant bone tumors do occur in horses, e.g., *multiple myeloma* (which is derived from *plasma cells*, whose function is to produce antibodies). Flat bones such as the spine, ribs, skull and pelvis are mostly affected with this disease. Bony changes resulting from multiple myeloma can be detected on X-rays, and the patient often exhibits back pain. Benign tumors (*osteomas*) affecting the flat bones of the equine skull, and *cartilaginous* benign tumors (*osteochondromas*) affecting the long bones (i.e., the legs) do not generally preclude chiropractic adjusting.

6. **Bone infections.** While these are rare, they still exist and should be ruled out by a veterinary medical examination. Some signs of bone infections are tissue atrophy, increased warmth, and *edema* (swelling due to fluid buildup). Sometimes a soft-tissue mass will be present that lacks roundness and changes shape under pressure. *Infectious arthritis*, for example, is a bacterial infection most commonly affecting the hock, carpus, stifle and fetlock; it is often seen in foals due to the spread of bacteria from the umbilical cord into the bloodstream.

7. **Nerve damage.** The sensation over these areas is usually decreased; therefore, the degree of susceptibility to injury cannot be adequately assessed.

8. **Old surgical scars,** especially on or near a joint. These are signs that the horse has had something wrong with it. Find out what it was before you adjust.

9. **Profuse joint swelling.** Large areas of increased heat and excess fluid are signs of a serious medical condition. A *sprain*, which is a tearing or stretching of a ligament (the "joint glue"), may be present, in which case the joint would be *hypermobile* or over-stretched and should not be adjusted.

10. **Skin lesions.** Adjusting over a lesion can aggravate the site and cause infections. Also, a skin lesion denotes a medical condition and should be immediately evaluated by a vet.

11. **Medications.** Pain killers and anti-inflammatory drugs such as phenylbutazone can mask symptoms—even though chiropractic care may help reduce the need for such medications. Side effects of medications (as well as some food supplements) may present themselves as subluxations, i.e., increased or decreased muscle tone over the spine.

12. **Herniated (slipped) disc.** I saved this for last as a reminder that horses rarely, if ever, suffer from herniated discs. Nonetheless, a slipped disc does preclude chiropractic manipulation.

CHAPTER 7

HANDLING & SAFETY

If you bought this book, you most likely own a horse (either that or you're hopelessly addicted to book buying). So assuming that you do own a horse, you should know your animal fairly well and vice versa, which means there shouldn't be too many safety worries. But performing equine chiropractic raises added handling and safety concerns. Applying a sudden thrust into a still animal can be unsettling and cause your horse to react unpredictably. Therefore, you must be prepared and take necessary precautions.

As sure as the Cubs will never win a World Series—dogs bite and horses kick. While you will always hear a dog owner say, "My dog doesn't bite,"* you will never hear a horse owner say, "My horse doesn't kick."

GENERAL SAFETY ADVICE

1. With any horse, do not approach him suddenly. Walk toward him within his field of vision, stop, and then start again. If you walk straight toward an animal, they perceive you as a predator. If you take your time

---

* This reminds me of the old *Pink Panther* routine. First man (having just been bitten): "But sir, you said your dog didn't bite." Second man: "That's not my dog!"

and retreat a little as you approach, they feel more at ease.

2. Do not make any sudden movements once you're next to the animal. Continually speak in a quiet, kind, but firm manner without any outbursts.

3. Brush your horse with the palm of your hand as opposed to patting him. Patting or slapping will either frighten your horse, or make him think you're giving him a command he doesn't immediately understand.

4. Approach the horse from his left side; they're more accustomed to this, since riders mount and dismount from this side. Also, if you're the practitioner, stand on the same side as the owner. If the horse gets nervous, he'll be looking for his owner for help and he'll see you there as well.

5. Horses can kick hard with their hind legs, especially when you are standing directly behind them. If you are in kicking range, stand close to the *side* of the horse's hindquarters, so that if he does kick you won't receive the full force of the blow.

6. Keep the immediate working area clear of any debris. A horse, for example, can step in an open chair or crate and break his leg.

7. During the adjustment, only you and your assistant should be contacting the horse. Keep onlookers to a minimum and out of range.

8. When picking up the front leg (foot), start by touching his shoulder, and for the hind leg, his hip. This is very important.

9. If you don't know how to lift up the front or hind leg, seek the advice of an experienced farrier or trainer. Generally, when picking up the front leg, tap behind the knee or pinch the flexor tendon (Fig. 7-1). The horse should respond by bending the knee. When picking up the hind leg, start by flexing the stifle (true knee), and lean into the horse

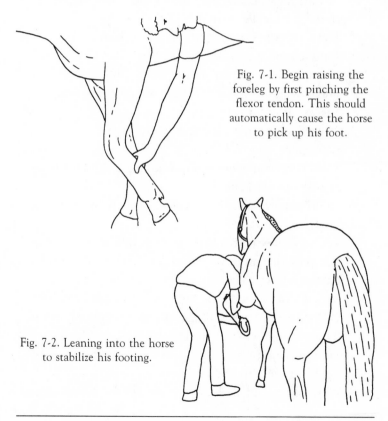

Fig. 7-1. Begin raising the foreleg by first pinching the flexor tendon. This should automatically cause the horse to pick up his foot.

Fig. 7-2. Leaning into the horse to stabilize his footing.

to stabilize his footing. Essentially, you become a temporary leg (Fig. 7-2).

10. While working around his head, sometimes it helps to gently blow into his nostrils. This helps you "bond."

SAFETY ADVICE DURING ADJUSTING

1. Always have an assistant control the horse's head, even during cervical adjusting.
2. For those methods requiring you to stand on a platform, use a firm but soft foundation, like a bale or two of hay. Chairs are dangerous and wobbly.
3. Never adjust in the stall. There is no place to escape in the event of an emergency.
4. Always adjust in a wide open area, like an arena or an open pen.
5. Make sure bystanders are not standing behind the horse during the adjustment.
6. If the horse is too rambunctious, do not adjust him that day.
7. For adjustments that require close head contact (e.g., the posterior atlas move), remember, head-butting is dangerous too. Keep your ear close to the horse's cheek, so you won't receive the brunt of a sudden head butt.
8. Do not use cross-ties, ropes, or chains while adjusting. Those things will hurt your horse if he decides to bolt after the adjustment. Instead, the assistant should maintain control with the lead.
9. Don't be afraid to be a coward. If the horse starts

acting wild after the treatment, get off the hay and escape, unless you have to assist someone else in trouble.

10. Keep other animals away during the adjustment. Dogs bark, and you can easily trip over them.

RESTRAINING TECHNIQUES

First, this sweeping statement: **Use as little restraint as possible.** Restraining a horse causes him to tense up and feel caged in, which in turn leads to muscle tension. Having to restrain a horse implies he's not cooperating. Instead of forcing him to cooperate, find out why he's acting skittish. Did something scare him? Are there too many people around? Did he recently suffer a bad experience? Is he on any medications? All of these questions must be answered before you attempt any restraining methods. Then you have to ask yourself if you want to adjust your horse badly enough to put both of you in danger. If the risks outweigh the benefits, just forget it. Adjusting should be a relaxing experience.

Here are some common types of restraining techniques. They were designed to keep the horse under control during routine body maintenance (shoeing, grooming, bandaging, etc.), where tense muscles really don't matter.

1. **Head collar, halter, and lead:** This is the best of all. If you can control the horse's head, you'll have control of the entire animal. Use of a head collar and lead is standard and safe, and horses are used to it (Fig. 7-3).

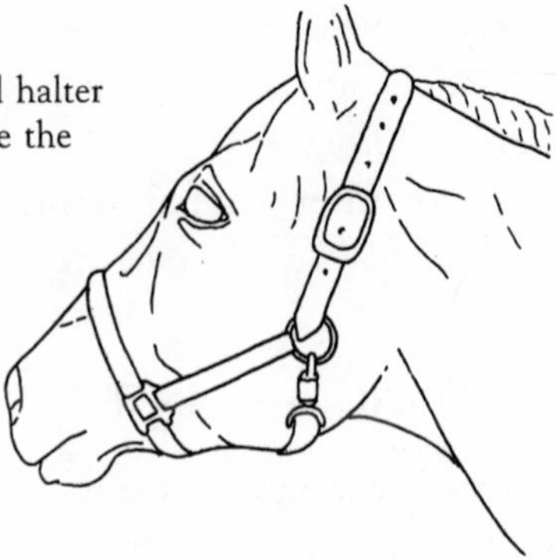

Fig. 7-3. The head collar and halter are used as handles to guide the horse's head.

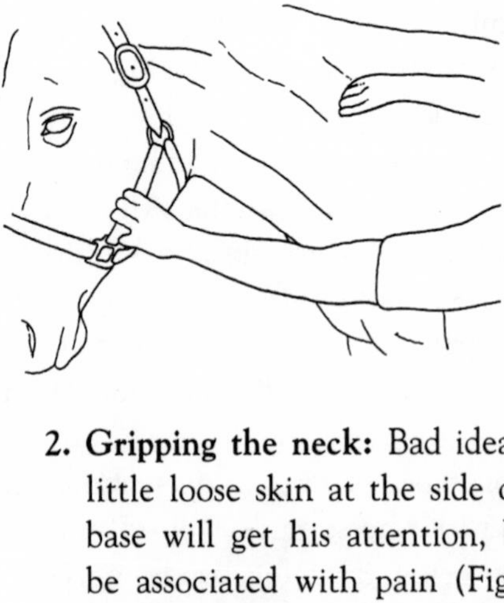

Fig. 7-4. Restraining your horse by pinching some loose skin at the side of his neck.

2. **Gripping the neck:** Bad idea, but quick. Pinching a little loose skin at the side of the neck towards the base will get his attention, but the adjustment will be associated with pain (Fig. 7-4).

3. **Ear twisting:** Even worse than skin pinching, but can be very effective during emergencies. To apply the ear twist, sneak up behind the ear from the back of the neck and grasp the entire ear with your hand (Fig. 7-5). Be careful not to grab at it. Apply slow, steady pressure—as hard as necessary without

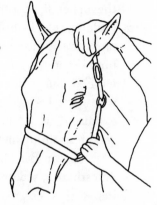

Fig. 7-5. Twisting your horse's ear will also restrain him. But use only in emergencies—horses hate this.

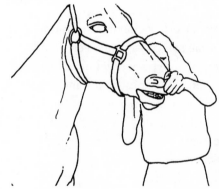

Fig. 7-6. Twitching your horse with your hand. Horses don't like this either, but it will get their attention.

hurting the ear. Try not to rely on this technique too often. Repeated ear twisting can make your horse head-shy.

4. **The twitch:** This is about as pleasant as the average root canal. But by twisting the upper lip with a metal twitch or similar devices (Fig. 7-6), you can successfully restrain a horse. Some horse handlers simply grasp a hunk of the upper lip with their hand and twist. It isn't fully understood why this restrains the horse, but some vets believe the acupuncture point contained in

the upper lip contributes to its effectiveness.

5. **Holding up a front leg:** By holding up a front leg, you prevent the horse from easily kicking you with the hind leg on the same side. This is not a bad restraining method, but it limits your adjusting techniques (e.g., you won't be able to adjust the hips, since hind leg extension would be impossible). However, this is a good restraining method while applying the Ligament Push (Logan Basic).

6. **Anesthetics, sedatives, or other chemicals:** Tranquilizers such as *acepromazine* can prove to be very handy, and will put the brakes on a hyperactive horse. I can't fault a vet for using them. But anesthetics and other chemicals are toxic to horses and are a leading cause of equine subluxations. Additionally, an artificially relaxed horse will lose natural muscle tone, rendering the adjustment less effective.

In conclusion, there is nothing more important than your *own* health. Delivering the adjustment takes a back seat to your safety, *no matter what*. Horses are bred and trained for man's use and enjoyment. A rowdy horse can wait another day for his treatment.

Nice Horsey!

In my first two animal chiropractic books, *The Well Adjusted Dog* and *The Well Adjusted Cat*, I included a section on the biting and least biting dog breeds, and on the more affectionate and more frisky cat breeds, respectively. I suppose the question here is which horse breed is more likely to kick or head-butt you. Which is the most challenging breed?

I personally think there's no such thing as a bad horse—only people who treat horses badly. But again, for what it's worth, here's a list of some trainers and horseman's opinions on which horses are more affectionate vs. more lively. Note: A horseman will often refer to a horse as being a "hotblood," "warmblood," or "coldblood." These monikers have nothing to do with the horse's body temperature (technically, all mammals are warm-blooded), but rather, denotes their origin and temperament. Arabians, for example, are hotblood horses which originated in desert climates such as Syria and Turkey and are known for their "light bones," quickness and short fuse. Conversely, Clydesdales are big, lumbering coldblood horses which originated in the forests of northern Europe, and are considered calmer. Warmbloods are horses with a mixture of both hot and cold ancestors, such as the Swedish Warmblood.

Affectionate and Good-Natured Horses

1. Clydesdale (tops the list of good-natured horses—gentle giants)
2. Morgan
3. Peruvian Paso
4. Hanoverian (enjoys working and is very quiet)
5. Trakehner
6. Pinto (most of the time—but they have their moments)
7. Paint
8. Appaloosa

9. Quarter Horse (loves to work with cattle!)
10. Shire
11. Percheron
12. Shetland Pony
13. Miniature horse
14. Welsh Pony

"Livelier" Horses

1. Arabian (the top of this list is a tie with my second choice)
2. Thoroughbred (along with Arabians, the most fun to watch—but don't stand behind them too long!)
3. Standardbred (all racing horses should be somewhat spirited)
4. American Saddlebred
5. Peruvian Paso (determined, stylish breed—but mostly good-natured)
6. Swedish Warmblood (could belong on either list)
7. Pinto (as mentioned above, they have their moments)

Chapter 8

Adjusting Skills

Herein lies the controversy: How much skill is required to deliver a safe, effective chiropractic adjustment? This boils down to who should be doing the adjusting, which is precisely the point of writing a [mostly] laymen's version of animal chiropractic methods.

A chiropractor goes to college for a minimum of six years to become a licensed chiropractic physician. During this period, he or she becomes skilled enough to conduct a clinical practice. So why don't we leave animal adjusting to the competent professional who has worked so long and hard to be able to deliver a proficient adjustment? The reason, of course, is because of the legalities concerning chiropractors adjusting animals. Many state laws prevent chiropractors from doing this because veterinarians have prevailed in getting laws made in their favor. Hence, it is up to horse owners themselves to apply safe equine chiropractic methods that don't require a fifth-degree black belt.

Since adjusting skills haven't changed much since the writing of *The Well Adjusted Dog*, the following is a repeat of the chapter bearing the same heading (with slight modifications).

Just as a pianist has to know how hard to press the key to create the right sound, the equine adjuster should develop certain sensitivities in their hands. There are two physical requirements for administering an adjustment: manual dexterity and muscular coordination.

Manual Dexterity

Traditional chiropractic moves rely on the mind and hand acting as one without hesitation. The movement your hands have to make during the adjustment is akin to the wrist action of cracking a whip, or to *Peanuts'* Linus "nailing" a fly out of the air with one quick snap of his blanket. It's speed, not force, that gets the job done safely. This is why an average-size person is able to adjust a horse—*without* the use of large hammers!

The adjuster should focus on developing a keen sense of touch and tactile depth perception. You should be sensitive to the subtle differences in muscle textures and heat variations. Some of the adjusting methods in this book involve applying light pressure, without having to actually deliver a thrust into a bone or joint.

Exercises to Improve Finger and Hand Skills

1. **Palpation exercise.** This will help to develop your sense of touch. Place a hair under a piece of notebook paper and see if you can feel the hair underneath. Then put the hair under two pieces of paper, and so on, until you're not longer able to feel the hair. If you can still feel the hair underneath five sheets of paper, you're above average.

2. **Testing finger depth perception.** Take a two-inch-thick piece of Styrofoam, hold it down with one hand

for stabilization, and place your other thumb on the Styrofoam's surface, keeping your wrist straight. This will be your adjusting hand.

Situate yourself above the Styrofoam with the elbow of your adjusting arm slightly bent. Now deliver a sudden impulse into the Styrofoam. Your thumb should not make a dent deeper than a quarter inch, even with a full and sudden thrust.

3. **Finger dexterity test.** With the palm of your hand on a table and your fingers slightly spread, place a quarter underneath the tip of your pinky. Then, without moving your pinky, slide your ring finger next to your pinky and pull the coin away, positioning it under your ring finger. Repeat this procedure for all your fingers, including your thumb. Then reverse the direction of the fingers. Do this until you can pass the coin from one side of your hand to the next in about five seconds.

Muscular Coordination

At the time of the thrust, your muscles must move in a clean, flawless motion. Your goal is to achieve bull's-eye accuracy.

Exercises to Improve Muscular Coordination

1. Practice driving a two-inch screw into a piece of wood without having to reinsert the screwdriver head.
2. Have someone throw three balls at you, one at a time in rapid succession. Catch and drop each ball with the same hand.

3. Toss two coins in the air and, with two separate grabs, catch them both.

General Advice

1. A horse is its own adjusting table. Therefore, it is safe to deliver an adjustment directly into the mid-back and lumbar vertebrae without supporting his belly underneath as is necessary with small animal adjusting.
2. For thrusting moves that deliver a sudden impulse into a joint, the force behind the thrust originates from the contraction of your triceps and pectorals.
3. For a "Set and Hold" adjustment, your hands remain at the end of the thrusting position for a few moments to prevent a recoil of the vertebra. This only applies after you've delivered a sudden impulse into a joint.
4. You do not always hear an audible "pop" during the adjustment. (The popping sound is gas escaping from a suddenly opened joint, and it has about a 20-minute refractory period, or the time needed to "refill" the joint with gas.) Sometimes you will simply feel the vertebrae slide into place. Whenever you do hear or feel a popping sound it is usually in the upper cervical or hip areas. Popping noises are generally not detected in the horse's thoracic area because the sound originates deep down in the vertebral joints, about a foot from the surface and buried within thick musculature.
5. If you want to adjust just one bone, you must contact only that bone. Contacting two bones divides the en-

ergy of your thrust in half.

6. The adjusting thrust is a high-velocity, low-amplitude (force) maneuver.

7. Even though speed is the primary component of the adjusting force, you do need some physical attributes, such as leverage, to deliver an effective adjustment. To maximize your own body's leverage and weight, you have to conform to the center of gravity. If you're standing on a bale of hay and hovering over your horse, make sure the top of your breast bone (sternal notch) is perpendicular to the heel of your hand (pisiform). This will allow you to thrust down and use a "body drop" all in one motion (Fig. 8-1). A "body drop" simply means your chest drops towards your contact hands during the thrust and is part of the momen-

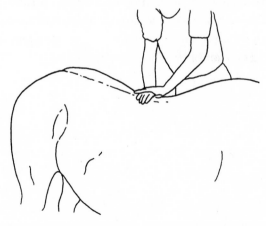

Fig. 8-1. While adjusting your horse's mid- or lower back, hover over your contact hand; this maximizes your body leverage.

tum. This is akin to having a strong wind at your back while running.

8. Both the practitioner and patient should be relaxed. I usually spend a few minutes getting to know the horse before the adjustment. Talking to your patient in a steady, soothing tone will help him to relax.

9. Try not to use too many restraints, since that leads to anxiety and muscle tension. Restraints could be too many handlers keeping the horse still, or drugs. Chemicals are toxic and can cause subluxations; use drug restraints (sedatives, anesthetics) *only* for safety reasons.

10. When indicated, remove all the joint slack before delivering the thrust. This is known as "taking the joint to tension." In the cervical region, this means to bend or flex the neck at the point of contact until it stops. In the mid-thoracic and lumbar region, removing joint slack means to push down into the vertebra and skin in the direction of the thrust until it stops.

CHAPTER 9

BEFORE THE ADJUSTMENT: MASSAGE & STRETCHING

If your horse needs to be adjusted due to musculoskeletal dysfunction, it means he's in pain. And pain implies that the muscles are sore due to taut and tender fibers, swelling (edema), and spasm. Maybe your horse has been through a bad time, such as an injury. If this is so, he needs to feel at ease. Muscles harbor stress, especially sore muscles.

There are several methods for treating the muscles, including massage, heat, cold, pressure points, trigger points, stretching, acupuncture, and of course chiropractic. Since delivering a chiropractic adjustment is the primary focus of this book, you should prepare your horse for the adjustment by gaining his confidence and letting him know you're there to help. The use of massage and relaxing the muscles prior to the adjustment will put both of you at ease. The art and skill required to effectively massage and stretch your horse cannot be explained in a few pages, so I'm not going to detail those techniques here. Instead, I'd like you to be familiar with a couple of stress reducing methods I use on my equine patients which make adjusting a whole lot easier. For further study on horse massaging, I highly recommend a book entitled *Equine Massage*, by Jean-Pierre Hourdebaight, R.M.T. (Howell Book House, 1997).

MASSAGING

Who doesn't like a good rubdown! Horses aren't much different from people in that respect. They have bigger muscles and, therefore, bigger needs. A tight muscle contains toxins, less blood flow, and decreased firing capabilities. Muscles need to be vital. They need to breathe. By applying digital pressure into a muscle, you can make this happen—fast!

Trigger Points

A *trigger point* is a painful, hard muscle derangement characterized by toxic build-up (lactic acid) coupled with decreased oxygen capacity. Horses get these from overexertion, and from not allowing the muscle to rest between activities. Trigger points feel like nodules and may vary in size. When stimulated with your finger, these sensitive areas will refer pain to other muscle areas. For example, a trigger point stimulated on the lower part of the neck may cause pain in your horse's shoulder, etc. Furthermore, these points follow a predictable pattern. A horse's inherent weaknesses usually remain the same throughout his life. In other words, a neck trigger point will always refer shoulder pain during times of stress.

To release a trigger point, simply apply and hold moderate finger pressure (2 to 5 pounds) into the nodule until it softens. This might take anywhere from just a few seconds to a couple of minutes. Your horse may react with pain at first, but will calm down once the point is relaxed. Equine massage therapists often recommend you first warm up a broad range of muscles surrounding the trigger points before treating the points themselves.

Muscle Squeezing

For chiropractic purposes, muscle squeezing is used along the entire back side of the neck and continuing down to the mane until the end of the withers, at which point the spines become flush with the body and can no longer be grasped. For maximum efficiency, grasp a muscle section with each hand as you're working down the neck (Fig. 9-1). Each squeeze should last no more than one second while applying about 10 pounds of pressure. Repeat this three times per session.

Compression

This is the massage technique you would use for the rest of the spine. If necessary, you may elevate yourself by standing on a bale of hay. Essentially, you are applying pressure to the spinal muscles with the palms of your hand (Fig. 9-2). Start your compression at the end of the withers and apply between 20 and 30 pounds in a pumping fashion—no longer than one second per pump—until you reach the base of the tail. This will stimulate blood flow and help break up muscle adhesions, thus making adjusting a much more enjoyable experience for you and your patient.

Elbow Technique

I learned about this technique early on in my equine adjusting career. Simply stated, you can direct much more pressure in one area with your elbow than with your hands (Fig. 9-3). This

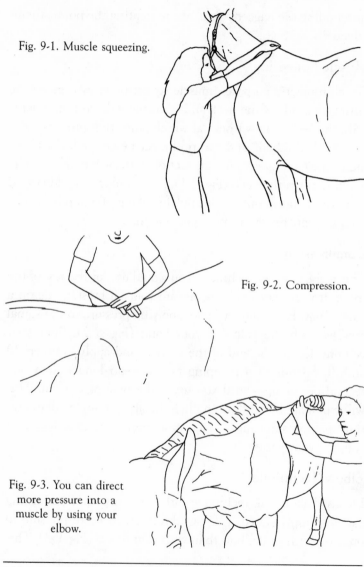

Fig. 9-1. Muscle squeezing.

Fig. 9-2. Compression.

Fig. 9-3. You can direct more pressure into a muscle by using your elbow.

main disadvantage of using your elbow is that it's awkward, especially if you're standing on a platform bending over your horse. The other disadvantage of using your elbow to massage muscles is the danger of applying too much pressure all at once and hurting your horse. You must be responsive and sensitive to his needs. Do not exceed 25 pounds of pressure, even on the largest muscles (i.e., the rump muscles).

STRETCHING

If you want to quickly release muscle tension in your horse's neck, shoulders, and leg, stretch each foreleg. Stand in front of your horse, grasp the leg below the knee, and pull his leg up towards you (Fig. 9-4). Hold this position for about 10 seconds and release. You can even stretch the foreleg backwards to further release foreleg and shoulder stress (Fig. 9-5). This technique can also be applied to the hind legs (Figs. 9-6a–b), but

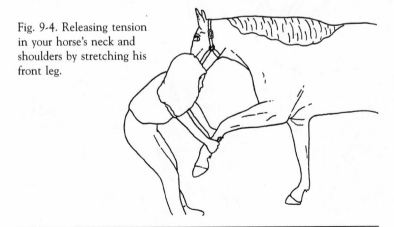

Fig. 9-4. Releasing tension in your horse's neck and shoulders by stretching his front leg.

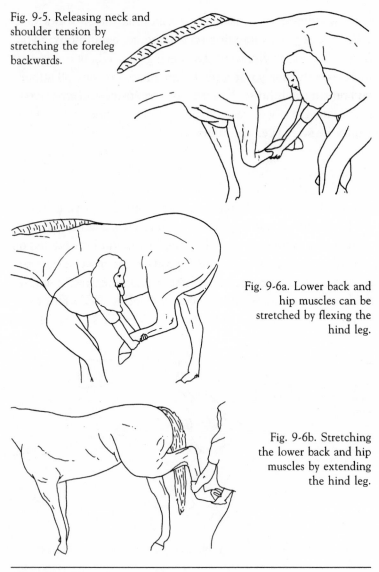

Fig. 9-5. Releasing neck and shoulder tension by stretching the foreleg backwards.

Fig. 9-6a. Lower back and hip muscles can be stretched by flexing the hind leg.

Fig. 9-6b. Stretching the lower back and hip muscles by extending the hind leg.

that can put you in danger of being kicked.

Stretching the back muscles can be accomplished by applying opposing forces with your hands (Fig. 9-7). It is helpful, but not always possible to stretch and isolate one muscle unless you are extremely adept in anatomy. However, by simply contacting a muscle section, applying opposite forces (e.g., traction to the right with your right hand and to the left with your left hand), and holding this "muscle traction" for about 10 seconds, you can release several tight muscle groups all at once. You can apply this stretching technique over several muscle groups as long as you don't exceed 20 pounds of pressure.

Incidentally, to get an idea of how much pressure you're capable of applying, sit on a chair, place a bathroom scale on a table, and push down into the center of the scale with one hand without using your body weight—just the force emitted from your arm and hand. You'll be surprised at how strong you are!

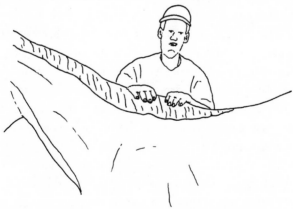

Fig. 9-7. Another way to stretch the back muscles: apply opposing force.

Other Therapies

In human chiropractic, the use of heat before an adjustment can be very helpful. The same applies with horses. Heat has an overall soothing effect on the nerves by improving circulation and facilitating oxygen and nutrients to the surrounding tissues. Many equine massage therapists recommend moist heat since it penetrates more deeply into the tissues.

Heat can be applied in many forms, but the temperature should not exceed 120 degrees Fahrenheit regardless of the heating method. If you want to adjust the mid-back, for example, you may apply heat by using a hot water bottle over the area for about 10 minutes. Heating lamps are effective, but impractical because you'll need electricity and a long extension cord, which can be dangerous if it gets tangled in the horse's feet. In my practice, I use *hydrocollator packs*, which are packs that contain mud and are preheated in hot water containers. These packs are very hot (about 160 degrees Fahrenheit) when they first come out of these containers, so I first wrap them in towels to lessen their intensity before setting them on my patient. Hydrocollator packs are safe to use because they eventually cool. Heat may also be applied with a hose dispensing hot water, or (in the best-equipped facilities) a warm-water whirlpool.

Cold is often used on horses following trauma to prevent excess swelling and to desensitize the skin or relieve pain. Ice packs, crushed ice wrapped in towels, and cold water from a hose are the most common methods of applying cold to a horse. I will sometimes use cold to reduce the horse's pain at a different site than the one I'm adjusting. For example, if the horse has an inflamed muscle over a lumbar area, he might not let me adjust his neck in fear that I'll somehow exacerbate his lower back pain. Applying ice to his lumbar inflammation will quell the pain there long enough for me to work on his neck.

As a chiropractor, I prefer to let the trainer, the vet, or other skilled employees administer heat or cold based on their recommendations and experience with their animal. However, I do administer the massage and stretching techniques myself. I feel this not only helps the horse's muscles relax, but also helps us relate to each other with a pleasant initial experience.

CHAPTER 10

NECK METHODS

Equine neck (cervical) adjusting is not only fascinating, it often yields dramatic results. By simply delivering one or two well-placed impulses, you can effectively reduce neck tension and joint fixations caused by weeks or months of stress due to riding, racing, training, etc.

The preceding chapters must be fully absorbed and reviewed before attempting the cervical techniques. Most students of this art will go through a few dry runs before administering the actual thrust. In chiropractic terms, a dry run is known as a *setup*. With a setup, all of the steps leading up to the adjustment will be followed except the impulse or thrust, which is the force needed to complete the adjustment. Deliver the thrust only when you feel confident of your abilities.

The next few pages describe five neck methods, which include three methods to adjust the atlas (first cervical), one special axis move (second cervical), and one method to adjust the rest of the cervical spine including the axis. For each method, you will be given a set of steps which must be followed each time in the sequence given. The steps will follow this order:

1. Static Palpation
2. Motion Palpation
3. Muscle Palpation

4. Setup
5. Thrust

Method 1: Atlas (Toggle Recoil)

The term *toggle recoil* is sort of a peculiar appellation for a chiropractic method, but descriptive nonetheless. The word *toggle* is defined as a verb, meaning to twist or turn, to manipulate a toggle switch, or to turn a switch (of an appliance, for instance) between two settings: "He *toggled* the TV between the baseball game and the news." *Toggle* is also a noun, commonly associated with electricity, such as a switch in which a projecting knob or arm, moving through a small arc, causes the contacts to suddenly open or close an electric circuit. Both of these definitions, in part, describe the action of the toggle recoil adjustment.

The term *recoil* means to coil again, or to spring back after discharging. So what does this have to do with the atlas?

The atlas is a ring-shaped vertebra which is different from all the others. The atlas has a less restrictive joint configuration than the other vertebrae and has the ability to oscillate within its own space when set in motion. Under slow motion video fluoroscopy, oscillation of the human atlas was demonstrated when a sudden thrust was applied on the atlas wing. The oscillation finally stopped, which resulted in re-communicating the cumulative body and brain's neural impulses by realigning the two holes together, i.e., the atlas ring with the *foramen magnum*, which is the opening at the base of the skull (see Chapter 3). Chiropractors often refer to this phenomenon of the atlas as "finding its own level." Its own level means the intended "slots," or where the atlas should be when it's not subluxated.

The reason why we use the word *toggle* with *recoil* is because as soon as you emit the impulse, your hand immediately comes off the contact (bone). This action is what allows for the oscillation. Compare this to a "set-and-hold" adjustment, where your hands stay at the point of contact for a few seconds after the thrust to *prevent* recoil. The recoil is the action of the elastic muscles snapping back at you once you've let go of it, like a slingshot.

Step 1. Static palpation: Feel each atlas wing at the side of the skull and determine if one of the wings feels larger, due to either a harder muscle mass or a misalignment. A misalignment would be present if the space between the atlas wing and the mandible (jaw bone) is smaller on one side compared to the other (see Chapter 4). The side with the smaller space is the side of the fixation or subluxation. The atlas, in this case, is not subluxated in relation to the mandible, but in relation to the base of the skull (occiput). The mandible is simply used as a guide to determine this. In other words, it is easier to feel the space between the atlas wing and mandible than between the atlas wing and occiput.

Step 2. Motion palpation: Stand in front of your horse, grasp both halters and extend his head up, then flex it down, and note if your horse resists this. If he does, check each side of the atlas by extending the head up and back to the right, back to neutral, then up and back to the left. Ask yourself which side felt "heavier" to extend. That would be the side of atlas fixation—usually the same side where you felt the smaller atlas-mandible space.

Step 3. Muscle palpation: Feel the muscles on each side of the atlas. The tighter muscle(s) implies joint fixation on that side, which should be consistent with your findings in steps 1 and 2.

Step 4. Setup: Stand on the side of the atlas wing fixation, contact the *cranial border* of that wing—the part of the wing closest to the base of the skull—with the pisiform bone in the heel of your hand (Fig. 10-1), and assume a fencer's stance. Next, have an assistant mirror your stance on the opposite side of the horse (Fig. 10-2). You have to be opposing each other exactly. If you're standing slightly in front of the horse's atlas, then your assistant is standing slightly behind the atlas. The

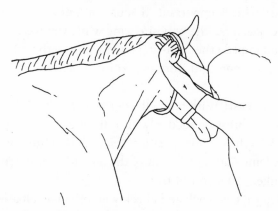

Fig. 10-1. Setting up for the toggle recoil. Contact the atlas wing near the base of the skull.

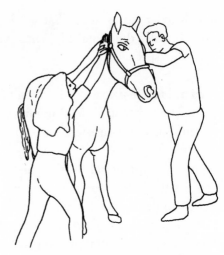

Fig. 10-2. During the toggle method, assume a fencer's stance (one leg forward, one leg back) for balance. The assistant opposes the practitioner, stabilizing the skull and the axis—but not the atlas!—on the opposite side of the head and neck.

only difference is that the assistant doesn't contact the opposite atlas wing; instead, he contacts the bone above (occiput or base of the skull) and the bone below (axis body or second cervical). This is important. If your assistant accidentally contacted or *stabilized* the opposite wing while you were thrusting, he would impede the adjusting force and stop the atlas motion entirely, preventing it from oscillating.

Step 5. Thrust: With your elbows somewhat bent, deliver the impulse by thrusting suddenly into the atlas wing, then recoiling back to the original position (Fig. 10-3). Think of Linus of *Peanuts* fame nailing a fly out of the air with one quick snap of his blanket. That sort of thing!

As always, go back and check your original palpation findings to see if the joint has been released. Note: Even after a successful toggle recoil, the space between the wing and man-

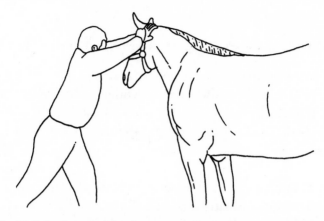

Fig. 10-3. In this example, the practitioner is taller, so his shoulder is more in line with the horse's atlas. This is preferable. If you're too short to reach the atlas adequately, have your assistant lower the horse's head to your shoulder level.

dible may still feel smaller, but if joint motion has improved, you're done.

Incidentally, there are some equine chiropractors that use this move exclusively, for *all* conditions, and have very successful practices. In fact, through most of the 1940s, the Palmer School of Chiropractic taught only this one technique (they now teach full spine adjusting). To some human chiropractors, the toggle recoil is the sole technique needed to harmonize the nervous system with the body and brain. They even use this technique to treat low-back pain! In my opinion, this thinking is antiquated. Personally, I have enjoyed better results by checking and adjusting the entire spine. Then again, people's opinions vary. That's why ice cream comes in chocolate, strawberry, and vanilla!

Method 1a: Atlas (Cranial Wing Move)

The cranial wing move is actually a variation of the toggle recoil move, without the recoil. Essentially what you're doing here is manually opening up the side that exhibits the smaller space between the atlas wing and the base of the skull (occiput).

Step 1. Static palpation: Same as for Method 1.
Step 2. Motion palpation: Same as for Method 1.
Step 3. Muscle palpation: Same as for Method 1.

Step 4. Setup: Stand on the side of the narrowed atlas/occiput space. If that space is closed on the left side of the horse, then grasp the halter with your left hand and contact the cranial portion of the atlas wing (Fig. 10-4) with your right pisiform. The cranial portion is that part of the atlas that is closest to the base of the skull (see Fig. 3-5b). Next, bend the neck by pulling the head toward you with your left hand.

Step 5. Thrust: Once the setup is complete, quickly thrust with your contact hand in two directions: caudally (toward the tail), and laterally (across the shoulders). Your stabilization hand (left, in this example) should be keeping the horse's head rigid. You don't have to withdraw your hands as swiftly as with the toggle, but the horse may ask you to stand clear, anyway. When the adjustment is complete, recheck your palpation findings.

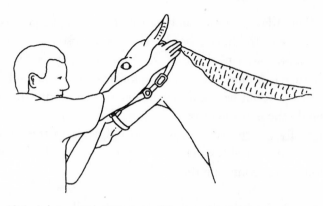

Fig. 10-4. Atlas cranial wing move. The practitioner is contacting the part of the atlas wing which is closest to the base of the skull (occiput). From the position shown here, he pushes the wing down caudally (tailward), while flexing the horse's head toward himself (not shown).

METHOD 2: ATLAS (POSTERIOR ARCH MOVE)

The names assigned to chiropractic methods are there to iden-tify some feature of the technique. In the first example, the term *toggle recoil* described the dynamics of the thrust. This next atlas method is called the *posterior arch move*, which de-scribes the part of the atlas which can be identified as mis-aligned in relation to the base of the skull. Therefore, the term "posterior arch," when both words are used together, means the actual named part of the atlas. When the term "posterior" is used by itself, it means the *direction* the dorsal/posterior arch of the atlas has subluxated. This is not as confusing as it sounds. But it is unfortunate that the direction of the subluxation and the anatomical part of the atlas are both termed "posterior."

The atlas' posterior arch can be felt right below the poll (the back of the horse's head). The word "posterior" is a term used more often to describe the back of a person than of a quadruped. A more accurate term for this move when referring to horses would be the *dorsal arch move*. The term "dorsal" is roughly the equivalent of "posterior." The only reason I don't originally use the term "dorsal" in reference to this move is because the mid-back vertebrae (thoracics) are *also* known as dorsals, thus confusing the reader.

Step 1. Static palpation: Providing you're tall enough, stand in front of your horse and reach around the back of his head with both hands to feel both sides of the atlas' posterior arch (Fig. 10-5). Review Chapter 4 if necessary. Your horse should be facing you in a relaxed, neutral position. This side that feels higher (towards the sky) is the posterior side.

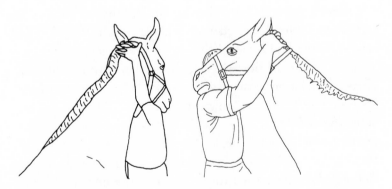

Fig. 10-5. Clasping your hands around the poll for the posterior arch move.

Step 2. Motion palpation: As in all atlas moves, check the "Yes" joint (see Method 1, Step 2). As you raise your horse's head up to the right and then left, notice which side offers more resistance. That would be the side of the posterior atlas. Verify this with the next step.

Step 3. Muscle palpation: Now that you've determined through motion palpation that one side was harder to raise up, let's say the right side, then feel the muscles over the right side of the arch and compare them to the left. If the muscles feel harder on the right, that means the muscles there are in spasm, thus fixing the right atlanto-occipital joint (the joint between the base of the skull and atlas) and pulling the arch up (posterior) on the right. A tight and spastic muscle on one side would explain why neck extension (as in Step 2) is more difficult on that side. The joint is fighting you.

Step 4. Setup: Stand in front of your horse on the side opposite the fixation or the high posterior arch. For a right posterior arch subluxation, stand on the left side of your horse with the horse's jaw resting on your left shoulder. In essence, your left shoulder becomes the adjusting table! Next, clasp your hands around the poll (see Fig. 10-5), contacting the whole atlas arch, with slightly more emphasis on the high arch side. (I think Edith Bunker on *All In The Family* used to say that. "Hi Arch!") Then, with an assistant stabilizing the front of the right shoulder (so the horse doesn't move forward), take one step backwards. This will extend and traction out the joints (Fig. 10-6). Next, move one short step to *your* right. This takes the joint to tension by

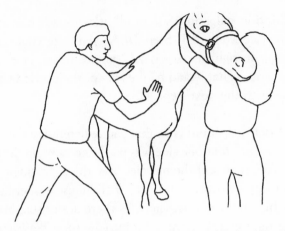

Fig. 10-6. An assistant stabilizes the horse near the shoulders during the posterior arch adjustment.

removing the "slack," and opens up the closed atlas/mandible side. **Note:** Horses often resist having their heads brought down and forward like this, and will buck their heads up. I regularly have to make two or even three attempts before the horse finally cooperates. A few years ago, a trainer taught me a neat little trick to relax the horse's neck before administering this move. She told me to simply grasp the poll and guide the head down until the nose touches the ground, and hold this position for about a minute until the neck muscles relax, then slowly allow the horse to raise his head.

Step 5. Thrust: Once all the setup steps are in place, then suddenly thrust down with both hands, with a little more emphasis on the right (fixed) side. Essentially, you are knocking the high (posterior side) down. Remember, speed is *everything!*

At least, I want you to think that. Speed more than force. More times than not, you will get an "audible" or joint popping with this move. Again, hearing a "pop" is not necessary to complete a successful adjustment (although most of my students would say I'm a slave to the audible!).

Important note: It is possible for the atlas to subluxate *straight* posterior, and be fixed (locked) on both sides. This is more of a subjective call when testing the "Yes" joint for the amount of extension. If, during motion palpation, your horse's head is difficult to raise (extend) up, then adjust the atlas accordingly without deference to a right or left fixation. You do this by following all of the setup steps except the last step which is taking a short step to your right (or left), then thrust straight down as in Step 5. This is merely a variation of the posterior arch move.

Method 3: Atlas (Anterior Wing Move)

This one sounds like something a bird would do after crashing into a window! In reality, the *anterior wing move* is a modification of the posterior arch move. It was originally designed to accommodate practitioners who are too short to clasp their hands around their horse's poll to perform Method 2. The idea is that the bottom (anterior or ventral) part of the atlas wing is lower and more accessible than the posterior arch. If this is true, then why not just skip Method 2 altogether and perform Method 3? The answer is that you have more control over the atlas with Method 2, since you're contacting more of the bone. Method 3 should be used only when Method 2 is impossible to

perform (the practitioner is too short, or the horse is too ornery—though not vice versa).

Step 1. Static palpation: Exactly the same as Method 2. Once
you know the side of the posterior arch, you know the anterior
wing is on the opposite side. Therefore, the anterior aspect of
one atlas wing would feel lower than the other. Think of it this
way: if you lower your right ear to your right shoulder, your
right atlas wing becomes much more anterior than your left.
The word *anterior* means in the "front" or abdominal plane—
the opposite of *posterior*. The word *ventral*, used more in veterinary circles, is approximately synonymous with *anterior*.

Step 2. Motion palpation: Again, exactly the same as Method 2.

Step 3. Muscle palpation: The same as Method 2, but keep in
mind that you're feeling for the tight muscles (posterior side)
only so you'll know where the less tight, anterior side would be.

Step 4. Setup: Using the method two example (right posterior/
fixed side), stand at the left side of your horse, which is the side
of the anterior (ventral) wing. With the heel (pisiform) of your
right hand, contact the anterior left wing (the part of the wing
closest to the horse's throat; Fig. 10-7). Then, with your left
hand, grasp the left halter and guide your horse's head down
(towards his chest). Next, take out the rest of the joint slack by
bending and turning your horse's head into the heel of your
right hand until the joint is brought to full tension.

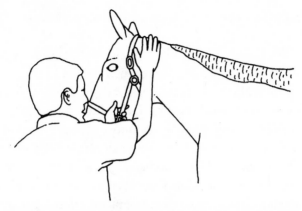

Fig. 10-7. Atlas anterior (ventral) wing contact. Begin the adjustment by placing the heel of your hand (pisiform bone) on the low (anterior) aspect of the atlas wing.

Step 5. Thrust: Once the setup is complete, quickly thrust up towards the posterior (high) arch—using only your contact hand (right hand, in this example) to deliver the thrust. Keep your left hand as solid and still as possible during the adjustment. In essence, you're pushing the low side of the atlas *up* as opposed to driving the high side down, as in Method 2. The key word here is speed. Your adjusting hand/arm must be quick, not forceful, to perform this move.

METHOD 4: AXIS (SPINOUS CONTACT)

This move is called the *spinous contact*, thus delineating the axis' special feature from the rest of the cervicals. The special feature is the prominent spinous process; the axis, or second cervical, contains the only palpable spinous process in the neck, which can be used as an adjusting contact point.

Step 1. Static palpation: When you look at an isolated picture of the axis, its spinous looks as though it would conspicuously project above the atlas, or the back of the neck. This is not the case. When palpated, the axis feels like a narrow, shelf-like ridge, hovering just below the posterior arch of the atlas. The only difficulty you might encounter during static palpation is not being tall enough to reach around the neck. If that is so, lower your horse's neck until it's level with your head. Note: The fundamental purpose of chiropractic spinous palpation is to determine the side of laterality, or the direction of the mis-alignment. Is the spinous off-center to the left or right? This question cannot be answered solely with static palpation. The bony spinous itself may be wrought with irregularities, such as bony calcium bumps, which would cloud your assessment. That's why the next step, motion palpation, is the main indicator of spinous laterality.

Step 2. Motion palpation: To determine axis spinous laterality, you must first ascertain the side of the neck to which the axis *body* has rotated. To do this, stand to one side of your horse's neck—the left, for example. Grasp the halter with your left hand, and place the heel of your right hand on the axis body by first feeling the left atlas wing, then dropping down below the wing and a little towards the throat (Fig. 10-8). You should feel the large, bulbous axis body there. Next, laterally flex (bend) the head into your contact hand as far as it will move. A horse's nose should point about 90 degrees to the horizontal (Figs. 10-

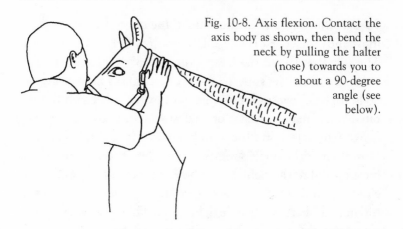

Fig. 10-8. Axis flexion. Contact the axis body as shown, then bend the neck by pulling the halter (nose) towards you to about a 90-degree angle (see below).

Fig. 10-9a. Bending the horse's neck towards you while contacting the axis body.

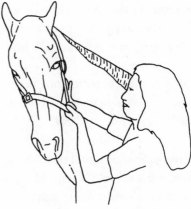

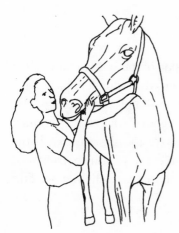

Fig. 10-9b. Bending the neck 90 degrees to the right. Note: You may contact the horse's chin or hold the halter to accomplish this.

9a–b). Now check the other side in the same fashion (switching hands, of course), and ask yourself which side bent *less*. The side that flexed the least is the side of axis body rotation. As an example, let's say it was the left side. The reason axis body rotation causes limited lateral flexion is because the rotated body creates a wedge or an obstacle between the vertebra above (the atlas) and the vertebra below (the third cervical). Now then, if the body is rotated on the left, the spinous had to have moved to the right, since the vertebra is all one piece. An easier example to picture is to give the "thumbs up" sign (à la Siskel and Ebert) with your right hand. The tip of your thumb represents the axis spinous; the fleshy part below your thumb represents the axis body. Then rotate your wrist to the right. Your thumb tip now points to the right, and the fleshy part has rotated up towards the left. Just that simple!

Step 3. Muscle palpation: With obvious axis-spinous laterality, you will be able to feel a harder muscle next to the side of the deviation (Fig. 10-10a).

Step 4. Setup: Stand next to the side of spinous laterality—the left, for example. Grasp the halter with your left hand, and with the heel of your right hand (pisiform bone: the "pointy heel" below your little finger just above your wrist), contact the axis spine (Fig. 10-10b). If you're too short to reach the spinous, lower your horse's head. Next, pull your horse's head towards you until it stops, and rotate his nose slightly up. This brings the joint to tension.

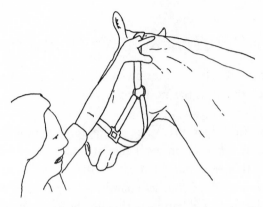

Fig. 10-10a. You will feel a harder muscle next to the side of axis spinous deviation.

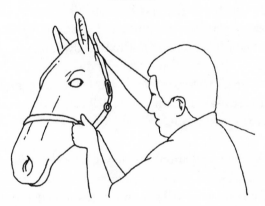

Fig. 10-10b. Contacting the axis spinous with the heel of your hand.

Step 5. Thrust: Once Step 4 is in place, sharply thrust right to left with your contact (right) hand. Note: Sometimes the bone will move just from setting up and taking the joint to tension. If this happens, you don't need to thrust.

Method 5 (Cervical Body Contact)

This method can be used for all of the neck bones except the atlas, since the atlas has no body.

Step 1. Static palpation: What you're doing here is feeling all of the cervical bodies on each side at once and palpating for the one(s) that stick out the most. To do this, stand in front of your horse and place your left hand on your horse's right axis body, and your right hand on the left body. Remember, the cervical bodies are situated more towards the throat and are far removed from the mane. Next, scan all the way down the neck, making sure you're contacting the same bone on each side (right and left sides of the axis body, for example). The prominent projections you'll feel along the way are the body's bony *transverses*. If, for example, you feel a more pronounced right transverse at the 5th cervical level, take note of that. That is probably the side of a 5th cervical body rotation.

Step 2. Motion palpation: Review Chapter 4. But for now, stand to one side of your horse, grasp the halter, and guide his head as far as his nose will go towards his shoulder. Repeat this on the other side. The side that bent the least should contain a rotated cervical body (as signaled by a more prominent transverse). This is the *passive* motion test, because your assistance is required. Next, utilize the *active* motion test by waving a fresh carrot under his nose and leading his head/neck towards each shoulder. If your passive and active findings are inconsistent, the active motion test supersedes the passive test. Once you know the side of least lateral flexion, isolate the exact rotated body by placing your hand on the more prominent transverse of the fixed side and comparing its motion to the other side.

Step 3. Muscle palpation: You should feel tighter muscles surrounding the rotated cervical body.

Step 4. Setup: As an example, let's say the 5th cervical body is rotated to the right. Stand next to the right side of your horse and contact the *lamina-pedicle junction* of the body (just dorsal to, or above, the transverse) with your left pisiform (heel of your left hand). Your right hand is busy grasping the halter and controlling your horse's head. Next, bend the head/neck towards you as far as possible to take the joint to tension. Next, rotate the nose up a little towards the sky. Your contact arm should be at a 45-degree angle to the vertical (Figs. 10-11a–b).

Step 5. Thrust: With your contact and stabilization hands in place, impulse suddenly in the direction of the opposite ear (which is approximately a 45-degree angle). You will sometimes hear or feel a "pop" with this move. As with most cervical adjusting, the bone may move from simply setting up the adjustment. If so, you don't need to thrust.

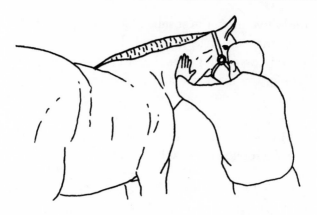

Fig. 10-11a. Setting up for a right cervical body contact.

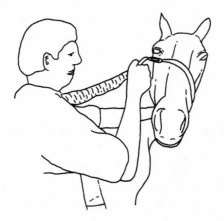

Fig. 10-11b. Bringing the horse's neck to tension for the
cervical body contact.

CHAPTER 11

MID~BACK (THORACIC) METHODS

To call the thoracic vertebrae the mid-back is stretching the truth a bit. There are 18 vertebrae in the equine thoracic (dorsal) spine, of which the first 8 or so are located in the upper back (the withers). The motion of the thoracic spine is limited compared to the cervical and lumbar spine, because each thoracic articulates with a rib on each side, which braces the back. It is because the ribs add rigidity to the back that horses are able to support a rider. You would think that this stiff configuration would prevent horses from getting subluxated here. It should, but doesn't because of two basic reasons: riders mount their horses from the left side of the animal, which pulls the thoracics down on the left; and saddles are frequently ill-fitted, which puts stress on the upper and lower thoracics. Other reasons the thoracics become subluxated include obese riders, riding a lame horse (due to foot and leg conditions), jumping, too much stall rest (getting stiff in the stall), and insufficient warm-up before activities such as racing, dressage, and training. Here are the three most commonly used thoracic methods.

METHOD 1: UPPER THORACIC TECHNIQUE

Since the first thoracic spinous is usually not palpable, the upper thoracic methods are for the 2nd through 8th dorsals.

Step 1. Static palpation: In the upper thoracics, you will be able to feel not only the spinous tips, but a small portion of the spinous sides. So place the fingertips of both your hands on each side of the second thoracic and slowly, but firmly, run your fingers down the withers until you reach the 8th dorsal (Fig. 11-1). Along the way, note which side feels lumpier in spots. These lumps would be a thoracic spinous poking through the muscles. Thus, a lump on the left side of the withers means that spinous has deviated to the left. Just like that! Also, check the muscles surrounding the scapula on that side. They, too, should feel tight compared to the opposite side.

Step 2. Motion palpation: Grasp the deviated spinous tip and try wiggling it back and forth, like a tooth. It will move (spring) less when you push it towards the opposite side of the spinous laterality.

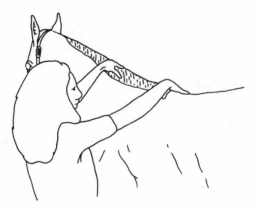

Fig. 11-1. Palpating the upper thoracic spinouses. This is the withers area, where the spinouses are most easily felt.

Step 3. Muscle palpation: As mentioned in the first step, you will feel tight muscles on the side of spinous laterality.

Step 4. Setup: Stand on the same side of spinous laterality. Place the heel of your hand (pisiform) on the spinous, just below its tip, while assuming the fencer's stance (Figs. 11-2a–b). Your other hand is placed over your contact hand. (Most practitioners are tall enough to reach this contact point without standing on a bale of hay). Make sure your arms are perpendicular to the contact and your elbows slightly bent. Next, have your assistant stabilize the horse by mirroring your image on the opposite side (Fig. 11-2b). Your assistant's hands should be pushing against the upper thoracics, but not on the bone you're about to adjust. He, too, should assume the girdered fencer's stance in anticipation of the impending adjusting force.

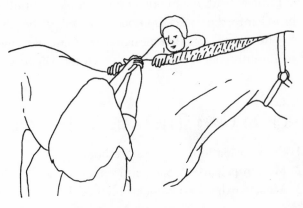

Fig. 11-2a. Upper thoracic technique. Ideally, your arms should be perpendicular to the spine (unlike this diagram). This picture shows the end of the adjustment, as the practitioner's arms are fully extended.

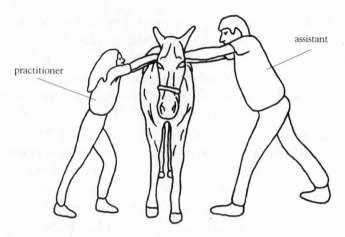

Fig. 11-2b. An assistant stabilizes the horse on the opposite side, ready to accept the force of the thrust.

Step 5. Thrust: With your contact hand in place, firmly push (not thrust) into the lateral spinous. This takes the joint to tension. Then, with a sudden motion, thrust lateral to medial, which is towards your assistant. Recheck your palpation findings.

Method 2: Upper Thoracic Variation

Step 1. Static palpation: Same as Method 1.
Step 2. Motion palpation: Same as Method 1.
Step 3. Muscle palpation: Same as Method 1.

Step 4. Setup: *Not* the same as Method 1! For this method, you are standing on the *opposite* side of spinous laterality, and no assistant is required (except maybe to hold the horse's head still). The idea of this technique is to *pull* the deviated spinous towards yourself, instead of pushing it away from you as in Method 1. Therefore, hook the middle and ring finger of one hand around the lateral spinous, with your other hand over it to support this arrangement (Figs. 11-3a–b). You don't have to assume the fencer's stance; rather, you should stand as close as possible to the horse.

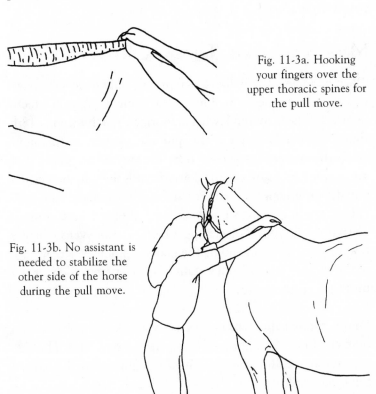

Fig. 11-3a. Hooking your fingers over the upper thoracic spines for the pull move.

Fig. 11-3b. No assistant is needed to stabilize the other side of the horse during the pull move.

Step 5. Thrust: Once your contact fingers are in place, take the joint to tension by pulling the spinous towards yourself until it stops. You may not notice any tension here by doing this, but you have to perform this step to make sure. Next, sharply pull (jerk) towards yourself and let go. Sometimes you will notice the bone slide into place, but you won't hear a popping sound since the origin of that noise is deep down near the bottom of the vertebra. Then, as always, recheck your palpation findings.

MID~ AND LOWER THORACIC TECHNIQUE

Once you leave the withers, you're only able to feel the very tips of the spinouses, which limits the number of possible techniques. But keep in mind, when adjusting the 9th through 18th thoracics, that the angle of the spinouses changes as you move down the spine. If you recall from Chapter 3, the upper thoracic spines imbricate (point) down towards the tail, then gradually straighten out until you reach the 16th thoracic (the anticlinal vertebra), which points towards the sky. As you move down from the 16th thoracic, the spinouses point ever so slightly towards the head—including the lumbar spinouses. Knowledge of the spinous angles is important once it's time to deliver the thrust.

Step 1. Static palpation: Palpate each side of the spinouses and note any muscular tightness. Compare the two sides. The side of a spinous exhibiting more muscle tightness is the side of spinous laterality.

Step 2. Motion palpation: While standing on a bale of hay, push down on each spine (from the 9th to the 18th thoracic) and determine which one springs less. That would be the subluxated vertebra. For the lower thoracics, you can test the motion of each spinous by grasping the base of the tail with one hand and pressing against each spinous with the heel of your other hand. Get a rhythm going (pull the tail–push the spinous, pull the tail–push the spinous) and test all of them within a few seconds. If the muscles resist this pushing, that would be the side of spinous laterality and the fixation.

Step 3. Muscle palpation: As mentioned earlier, the side of the spinous that displays the most muscle tightness is the side of the spinous laterality.

Step 4. Setup: Stand on a bale of hay on the same side as the deviated spinous. Contact the lateral spinous with the heel of your hand (pisiform), supported by your other hand (Fig. 11-4). Make sure your elbows are slightly bent so you have something to "spend." Maximize your body leverage by hovering over your contact hand so the top of your breast bone (sternum or sternal notch—the bony indentation below your throat) is perpendicular to the contact (Fig. 11-5).

Step 5. Thrust: Take the joint to tension (remove joint slack) by pushing—without thrusting—down and in line with the angle of the spinous, imbricated or non-imbricated, as the case may be. For adjusting purposes, your arms essentially become an extension of the spinouses. The reason for this adjusting

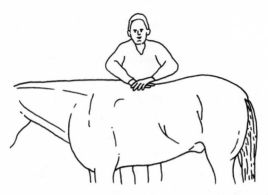

Fig. 11-4. Contacting the mid-thoracic spinous with the heel of your hand, which is supported with your other hand.

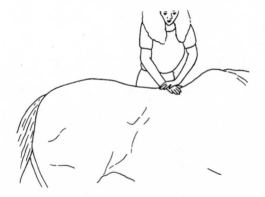

Fig. 11-5. Maximize your body leverage by hovering over your contact hand.

angle is to complement the joint facets (see Chapter 3), which decreases the friction of the joint below and makes your thrust much smoother.

Now, once the joint is taken to tension, deliver a sudden thrust with these three directions in mind: down towards the ground (dorsal to ventral), lateral to medial (from the outside to the center), and in the direction of the spinous (if the spinous points towards the tail, you want to thrust the spinous towards the head, etc.).

There is one notable variation of this adjustment. It is possible to stand on the opposite side of spinous laterality, make your contact by hovering a little further over the horse, then push the lateral spinous *towards* yourself. In my opinion, I find this variation somewhat awkward, since it's more difficult to maintain my balance on the bale of hay. But I use it anyway if I'm adjusting other vertebrae on that side and too lazy to get off the hay and lug it around the horse.

CHAPTER 12

LOWER BACK (LUMBAR) METHODS

The lumbar spine is susceptible to subluxations because of its relatively high degree of movement, especially at the transitional region where the last thoracic articulates with the first lumbar (thoraco-lumbar junction). Race horses who make wide turns on the track are particularly prone to low back subluxations, because they twist their backs at high speeds as they're rounding the turn.

As a group, the lumbars have no distinct curve such as a natural lordosis or hollow, which is a feature of bipeds (humans). The thoracic spine blends seamlessly with the lumbars much like two straightaway sections of track from a Lionel train set. Therefore, you have to be alert while palpating down the thoracics as you transition into the lumbars. The principal anatomical landmark demarcating this transition is the last pair of ribs which articulate with the last thoracic on each side. Once you feel the last rib on one side (just in front of the flank), you'll be able to trace its angle most of the way to the midline of the back, and approximate the rest of the angle up to the last thoracic. The next few pages describe the four most commonly used equine lower back adjusting methods.

Method 1: Lumbar Spinous Contact

Much like mid- and lower thoracic adjusting, you may use the spinouses to adjust the lumbars. Upon palpation, you will note that the lumbar spines feel somewhat sturdier and thicker than those of the thoracics.

Step 1. Static palpation: With lumbar static palpation, you again check for spinous laterality. To determine the direction of a deviated spinous, you must use reference points as a means of comparison. With thoracic static palpation, you compared the tightness of the muscles on each side of the spinous, with the tighter muscle being the side of the laterality. This also will work for the lumbars. However, the lumbars come equipped with extra anatomical projections, the mammillary processes, which can be palpated to determine the lumbar misalignment. Note: The last couple of thoracics also contain mammillary processes, but theirs are short and difficult to palpate.

Palpate from the sides of the first lumbar spinous all the way down to the last one. If you feel an obvious bump along the way, that's probably a high or protruding mammillary. This means the *body* of the vertebra has rotated up on that side, and its spinous (which is felt about half an inch or so down, caudal to the mammillary) has deviated to the opposite side. Thus, a high right mammillary means a left lateral spinous (Fig. 12-1).

Step 2. Motion palpation: Raise yourself above your horse by standing on a bale or two of hay. Place the heel of your hand

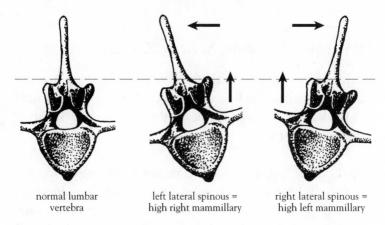

| normal lumbar vertebra | left lateral spinous = high right mammillary | right lateral spinous = high left mammillary |

Fig. 12-1. The relationship between a high mammillary and a deviated spinous. (Caudal views shown—your right = the horse's right.)

on a lumbar spinous and firmly, but not forcefully, push down (Fig. 12-2). As you do this for each spinous, you should notice a certain buoyancy or springiness which is a sign of normal joint motion. Any fixed or "dead" spots should be noted. Next, grasp the base of the tail with one hand, and place the heel of your other hand next to the first lumbar spine. Pull the tail and push each lumbar spine in a steady rhythm. The surrounding vertebrae should start to bend around your hand; if, instead, your horse resists this motion, the area that resists is the site of the fixation. You may also test lumbar motion by offering your horse a carrot and having him bend his neck to his shoulder (Fig. 12-3). During this test, you should notice a slight lift in his lower back. If your horse refuses to work for the carrot and won't bend his neck to one side, that could spell lower back pain, or back pain in general.

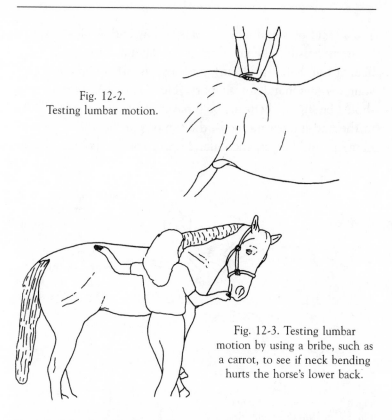

Fig. 12-2.
Testing lumbar motion.

Fig. 12-3. Testing lumbar
motion by using a bribe, such as
a carrot, to see if neck bending
hurts the horse's lower back.

Step 3. Muscle palpation: Taut and tender muscle fibers *directly*
to one side of a spinous indicate the side of spinous laterality. I
emphasize "directly" to distinguish these muscles from the fibers surrounding the mammillary processes, which are located
about half an inch in front of (cranial to) the spinous.

Step 4. Setup: Stand next to your horse on the side of the
spinous laterality; I'll use a left lateral spinous as an example.

You should be standing on a bale of hay and as close to your horse as possible. Next, contact the lateral spinous with the heel of your hand (pisiform), placing your other hand on top of your contact hand for support (Fig. 12-4a–b). Your elbows should be slightly bent so you'll have something to "spend." As in the mid-lumbar methods, the top of your breast bone (sternum) should be perpendicular to your contact point to maxi-

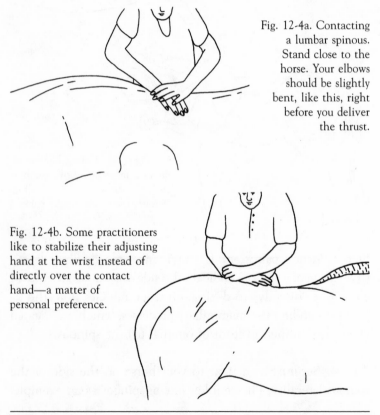

Fig. 12-4a. Contacting a lumbar spinous. Stand close to the horse. Your elbows should be slightly bent, like this, right before you deliver the thrust.

Fig. 12-4b. Some practitioners like to stabilize their adjusting hand at the wrist instead of directly over the contact hand—a matter of personal preference.

mize your body leverage. Then, firmly push your contact down towards the ground (ventrally) and in towards the midline— *without* thrusting. This brings the joint to tension (removing joint slack).

Step 5. Thrust: With your contact hands in place and the joint taken to tension, deliver a sudden thrust with your hands, bent elbows, shoulders, and body all working in unison. The thrust resembles an exaggeration of the motion a paramedic uses to start someone's heart while he's pushing on the chest during CPR. After you deliver the adjustment, recheck your palpation findings.

METHOD 2: LUMBAR MAMMILLARY CONTACT

The mammillary process is used when you don't want to use a spinous contact. It's a matter of personal preference; Methods 1 and 2 accomplish the same thing. You choose one method as a matter of convenience. If you're standing on the side of the high mammillary, you would adjust that mammillary, as opposed to the spinous which would be pointing away from you. With a mammillary contact, you're adjusting vertebral body rotation as opposed to spinous laterality.

Step 1. Static palpation: Same as Method 1.
Step 2. Motion palpation: Same as Method 1.

Step 3. Muscle palpation: *Almost* the same as Method 1 with one exception: When you feel a hard muscle knot right next to the spinous, that would be the side of spinous laterality. If you feel a hard muscle knot in front (cranial) and a little further out (lateral) to the spinous, that would be the high mammillary—which feels like an even harder muscle since there's bone underneath. Also keep in mind that the mammillary processes are shorter, thus, deeper than the spinouses. So you'll have to dig a little deeper to feel them.

Step 4. Setup: Stand on a bale of hay on the high mammillary side. Contact the high mammillary with the heel of your hand (pisiform) and place your other hand over the first hand. With slight elbow bend, hover over your pisiform contact with the top of your breast bone (sternal notch) perpendicular to the contact (see Figs. 12-4a–b). With both hands, firmly press down (ventral—towards the abdomen) to take the joint to tension. You are not thrusting here, just removing joint slack.

Step 5. Thrust: With your setup complete, deliver a sudden thrust straight down (towards the ground). As your elbows impulse down, your own body should drop some, to aid the momentum.

METHOD 3: LUMBAR LEG EXTENSION METHOD

This method is very similar to the first two, with one added step—an assistant raises and slightly extends one of the hind legs. The purpose of this step is to traction out the lumbars which allows more space for the vertebrae to slide during the adjustment.

Step 1. Static palpation: Same as Method 1.
Step 2. Motion palpation: Same as Method 1.
Step 3. Muscle palpation: Same as Method 1.

Step 4. Setup: Here's the difference. For a lateral spinous contact, stand on the side of spinous laterality, and setup as you would in Method 1. Have your assistant raise and extend the hind leg *opposite* of you (Fig. 12-5). In theory, extending the leg helps to open up the disc joints which adhere to the vertebral bodies. Extending the left leg, for example, helps to traction out more of the left disc (body) space. Therefore, when you push the spinous from right to left, the left lumbar body will adjust more easily due to the bigger slot. **Caution:** Extending a horse's hind leg can be dangerous. Horses can kick, bolt, or become off-balance. Only someone very experienced in this

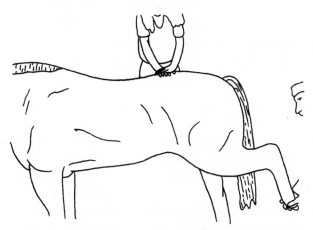

Fig. 12-5. The lumbar leg extension method. By extending the leg, you help bring the joints to tension.

procedure, such as a farrier or trained horseman, should assist you (see Chapter 7: Handling and Safety).

For a mammillary contact, stand on the side *opposite* the high mammillary (i.e., if it's on the horse's right, you stand on the horse's left). Then have your assistant raise and extend the hind leg opposite of you (hence, in this example, the horse's right). Standing on the side opposite the high mammillary is contrary to Method 2. But there's a reason: you should avoid standing on the same side as your assistant. Otherwise, you'll get in each other's way. Therefore, when contacting the high mammillary, you'll simply have to hover over your horse a little further to make your contact.

Step 5. Thrust: For both the spinous and mammillary contacts, apply the thrust at the height of leg extension. After delivering the force, quickly step off the platform while your assistant guides the leg back to the square position. Note: The horse should remain still. If the horse tries to walk, his back muscles will tense, making adjusting impossible.

METHOD 4: LUMBAR TAIL PULL

This is more of a general low-back stretching technique than an adjustment. It is widely used by trainers to increase their horse's flexibility before a race.

Step 1. Static palpation: Same as Method 1.
Step 2. Motion palpation: Same as Method 1.

Step 3. Muscle palpation: Once you know the side of spinous laterality, see if you can detect further spasms on that side.

Step 4. Setup: Stand on the side of the deviated spinous, the left, for example. Next, grasp the base of the tail with your right hand. With the heel (pisiform) of your left hand, contact the lateral spinous. Pull your horse's rear towards you with his tail (Fig. 12-6). This opens and tractions out the opposite side (right lumbar bodies) and removes joint slack on the lateral spinous side. As you're doing this, the lumbars should slightly bend around your contact hand.

Step 5. Thrust: You might feel the bones slide or "pop" by simply setting up. If so, you don't need to thrust. Rather, hold your setup for about 30 seconds, then release. However, if you think the vertebra needs to be adjusted, apply a quick thrust lateral to medial (out to in) while you're pulling the rear with the tail.

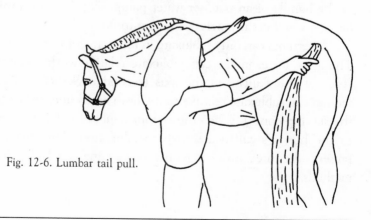

Fig. 12-6. Lumbar tail pull.

CHAPTER 13

SACRUM METHODS

Speaking as a chiropractor, if I had to name the two most strategic healing points of the spine, I would have to say the atlas and the sacrum. The atlas is important because it is the final barrier that simultaneously separates and links the body to the brain, the organ where all of the body's neurological impulses are processed. From a mechanical standpoint, the sacrum is the bone which stands guard to the rest of the spine. A subluxated sacrum can cause lower back pain, neck pain (via muscle compensation), an irregular gait, and loss of muscle power to the legs. Fortunately, the sacrum is easy to palpate and adjust. Its triangular shape and well-defined tubercles form a convenient lever at the end of the spine that can be likened to the handle of an outdoor water pump. By pressing on this handle, you'll get the nervous system to flow.

A vertebra can only subluxate in relation to another bone. The atlas, for example, can subluxate relative to the occiput (base of the skull) and the axis (second neck bone). The sacrum can subluxate relative to the last (sixth) lumbar and to the *ilia* (hip bones). When the sacrum is subluxated in relation to the hip, it's called a *sacroiliac* subluxation. This chapter presents the three most commonly used equine sacral adjusting methods.

METHOD 1: SACRAL PUSH TECHNIQUE

The name of this method says it all. You will be pushing down the high side of the sacrum. A sign of a high sacrum is when you're watching your horse walk straight away from you and notice that one hip hikes up higher than the other. The horse is attempting to take pressure off the sore leg or hip. People do this too—in a word, we limp. Sufferers of sciatica (pain down the hip or leg) will raise the painful limb as their foot strikes the ground. The hip that rises up would be the site of the high (posterior) sacrum.

Step 1. Static palpation: Stand to the side of your horse near the rump. Most people can do this while standing. Next, place the palm of your hand on the lower lumbar area and firmly feel your way down the back until you reach the summit of the hips. The hips' summits, the *tuber sacrales* (a.k.a. PSIS's; see Chapter 3), are the highest parts of the hip (one for each ilium, or hip bone), which are separated by a crevice. Underneath this crevice is the first sacral tubercle, which is equivalent to a vertebral spinous. Since the first sacral tubercle is somewhat buried under the tuber sacrales, it is not always palpable. However, the remaining four sacral tubercles are palpable. Thus, the sacrum spans from the tuber sacrales to the base of the tail. Now, feel the length of the sacrum and determine which side feels higher; that is the subluxated side.

Step 2. Motion palpation: What you're testing here is the motion of the sacrum in relation to the hips (sacroiliac joints). Place the palm of one hand over the tuber sacrales and your other palm on the second-to-last (4th) sacral tubercle, which is near the base of the tail. As you press down (towards the ground) on the 4th tubercle, you'll be able to feel the tuber sacrales "rock" up and down. Determine which tuber sacrale rocks the least. This is the side of the fixed sacroiliac (SI) joint. The high side of the sacrum is usually the side of the fixed SI joint since a high sacrum acts to close that joint, which is also splinted by tight muscles.

Step 3. Muscle palpation: Simply feel the musculature on each side of the tuber sacrales and determine which area feels harder. That harder side would be the side of the fixed SI joint.

Step 4. Setup: You will need to stand on a platform (a bale or two of hay) for this procedure. Stand next to your horse on the side of the high sacrum and place the heel of your hand (pisiform) on the high sacral tubercle. Next, while maintaining firm pressure on this tubercle, slide your pisiform off to the high side. Support your contact hand with your other hand (Fig.13-1).

Step 5. With your setup in place, firmly press the sacrum (without thrusting, at first) down towards the ground and slightly to the opposite side (medially or inward). This will take the SI joint to tension. Once this is in place, deliver a sudden thrust and immediately release your hands. Recheck the motion of the SI joint.

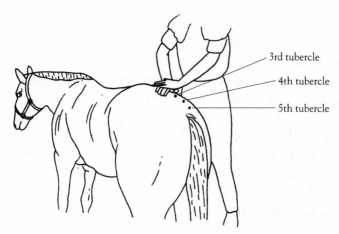

Fig. 13-1. Sacral push technique. Contact the high side of the sacrum. The diagram shows the practitioner contacting the second tubercle, but you may contact any of the high tubercles.

METHOD 2: SACRAL TAIL TECHNIQUE

Trainers love this move. Right before a race, they'll apply this technique to their horse to help free up the nerves to the lower back and legs. Then watch him go! It's almost unfair that not all trainers know how to do this.

Step 1. Static palpation: Same as Method 1 (feel for the high side).

Step 2. Motion palpation: Same as Method 1.

Step 3. Muscle palpation: Same as Method 1.

Step 4. Setup: This is as simple as it gets. Stand next to your horse on the high side of the sacrum. Generally, you won't need to stand on a platform. Next, grasp the base of the tail with one hand, and place the heel (pisiform) of your other hand against the 4th sacral tubercle. As you pull the tail towards you, push the sacrum away from you until you get a tight hold. This takes the SI joint to tension.

Step 5. Thrust: Before you thrust, hold your setup for about 30 seconds. This will provide some traction to the joint. After this time is up, thrust in the direction across the back and a little towards the head (Fig. 13-2). Hold the tail firm. **Thrust ONLY with your contact hand.** Then release.

METHOD 3: LIGAMENT PUSH (LOGAN BASIC)

This is one of the most effective equine chiropractic methods for helping rear leg lameness (providing the legs and feet are normal), hindquarter muscle weakness, and low-back pain. It is

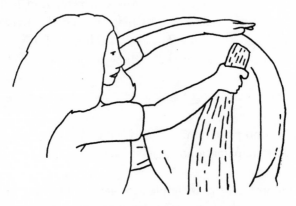

Fig. 13-2. Sacral tail technique.

also an excellent technique for instantly relaxing a stressed-out animal, providing you're able to stand behind him without getting kicked.

The Ligament Push is considered a sacrum adjustment even though you are actually contacting the *sacrotuberous ligament*, which is a broad ligament spanning from the sacral apex and first two tail bones (caudal or coccygeal bones) to the *ischial tuberosity* (Fig. 13-3; see also Fig. 3-18, p. 53). Hence the name "*sacro-tuberous.*"

You can liken the relationship the sacrum has with the sacrotuberous ligament by thinking of a hot air balloon. The sacrum represents the balloon and the ligament represents the strings. By pulling (or in this case, pushing) on one of the strings, you can effectively guide the direction of the balloon. The horse's head represents the wind currents, which usually have a mind of their own. As you'll soon see, you can control that, too!

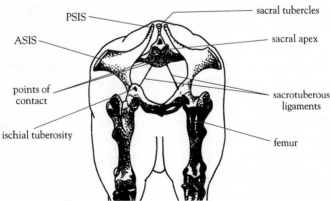

Fig. 13-3. Caudal view of the pelvis and the Ligament Push contact.

The Ligament Push, in my opinion, is more effective on animals than people, for two reasons. First, you have more direct control of the spinal cord by applying the Ligament Push in an animal because the cord ends further down the spine. In a person, the spinal cord ends at about the first or second lumbar. A horse's spinal cord ends at about the second sacral tubercle. Therefore, by applying a light force to the sacrum, you can take more stress off the spinal cord and help to balance the delicate pressure of the *cerebrospinal fluid* (CSF). This fluid is found in the ventricles of the brain, and between the spinal cord coverings (*arachnoid* and *pia mater*) known as the *meninges*. CSF helps cushion the brain during times of trauma, and also serves a metabolic function by acting as a medium for the transport of metabolites and nutrients between the brain and the blood. A fairly common viral disease of the meninges which causes fever, headaches, and stiff neck and back muscles is called *meningitis*.

The second reason the Ligament Push is more effective in animals is because it can be used more often in animals without fear of social consequences. Let me explain. This technique, for reasons soon to become apparent, is sarcastically known as "the brown thumb technique." But only if you're clumsy! The actual point of contact is near the anus. The person who is the recipient of this method lies face down on a chiropractic table with their pants pulled down past their waist. The doctor then finds the contact point and delivers the adjustment. This is all fine and dandy if your patient is well informed and isn't too modest. But there have been cases where competent chiropractors (usually a male chiropractor working on a female patient) have mistakenly been accused of taking unwanted liberties. A horse has never accused me of making unwanted advances because I usually buy them dinner first.

Step 1. Static palpation: Review static palpation for Method 1. Also, feel for the tight and painful sacrotuberous ligament. To do this, stand directly behind your horse (if he's not in a kicking mood), and draw the tail up (Figs. 13-4a–b). **Important safety tip: Horses are less likely to kick if you raise the tail as high as possible during the treatment. Also, to further assure**

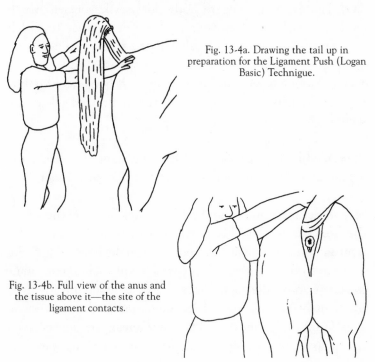

Fig. 13-4a. Drawing the tail up in preparation for the Ligament Push (Logan Basic) Technigue.

Fig. 13-4b. Full view of the anus and the tissue above it—the site of the ligament contacts.

your safety, construct a barrier by placing one or two bales of hay between you and your horse while performing the Ligament Push. There are two contact points: right and left. To palpate the right sacrotuberous ligament with your thumb, locate a point approximately 1:00 to the anus and apply light pressure up and in towards the center to feel the tip or *apex* of the sacrum (Fig. 13-5). If you move your thumb back and forth, you'll be able to feel a tough, fibrous cord, which is a section of the ligament. Feel its left counterpart approximately 11:00 to the anus (Eastern Standard Time!), and compare both sides. Ask yourself which cord feels tighter. Does your horse react to your touch? If you sense pain on one side, that is the side to adjust.

Step 2. Motion palpation: Review motion palpation for Method 2. The Ligament Push is applied to the high, fixed side of the sacrum.

Step 3. Muscle palpation: Feel for tight rump, low-back, and leg muscles. This would also be the side of your contact.

Step 4. Setup: Stand behind your standing horse on the side of the fixed sacrum. You'll be using a thumb contact. To treat the right sacrotuberous ligament, pose your right hand as if you're about to throw a football. This position will enable your thumb to scoop under the sacral apex. Next, contact the involved ligament by tucking your right thumb under the right sacral apex (1:00 to the anus), and fan your remaining fingers along the rump so they're pointing towards your horse's right ear and

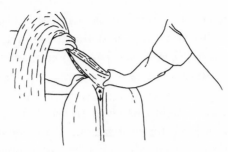

Fig. 13-5a. For the Ligament Push, first place your thumb at "12:00" to the anus, then slide over to "1:00" for a right contact or "11:00" for a left contact. Note: Pose your hand as if you're about to throw a football. This allows your thumb to scoop under the sacral apex.

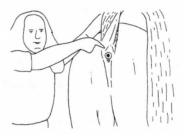

Fig. 13-5b. Ligament Push *left* contact point ("11:00").

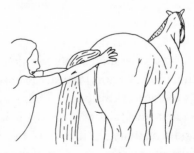

Fig. 13-5c. Ligament Push stance for a *right* contact. Note that the practitioner's fingers are directed toward the horse's right ear.

shoulder (Fig. 13-5c). Your contact arm should be straight and in line with your wrist and thumb, as if to form one solid cane. For now, your left hand should contact the left rump for stabilization purposes.

Step 5. Thrust: Initially, there is no thrust. What you're doing is applying *light* force to the ligament. The amount of force necessary for an effective adjustment is the maximum amount of pressure you can apply over your eyeball *without* hurting your eyeball (about 3 ounces of pressure). Maintain this pressure in accordance with your hand and thumb placement for about two minutes. During this time, massage all of the surrounding rump (gluteal) muscles, the muscles surrounding the lumbar spines, and the thigh muscles. Have your assistant massage the muscles surround the thoracic spines, and cervical muscles. Relaxing the upper cervical muscles is an important part of "directing the wind currents," as mentioned earlier. Once you relax a horse's neck muscles, he'll sigh with relief, drop his head, and become more controllable. At the end of the two minutes, deliver a final thrust (a light, quick "punch") in the same direction as the light force. Recheck your findings.

The Ligament Push can be used as often as four times a week (about every other day). Do not, I repeat, do *not* use a pencil or any other object to contact this point. They can be dangerous as well as misguiding since you wouldn't be able to accurately judge pressure and sensitivity. Incidentally, if you do not attain your desired results, change the direction of the force by aiming more towards the center of the occiput (base of the skull).

I am often asked if you can hurt your horse if you contact the wrong side. The answer is no. This technique is so gentle, the only consequence would be not getting the desired result. In other words, contacting the wrong side may simply prove ineffective.

The next chapter describes methods to adjust the pelvis. These techniques are just another way of adjusting the sacroiliac joint.

CHAPTER 14

PELVIS METHODS

The terms *pelvis* and *hip* are often used as synonyms. In everyday speech, this may be acceptable, but there are more than subtle differences. The pelvis is a basin-shaped cavity in the lower part of the trunk of most vertebrates. In the horse, the pelvis consists of the *ilium, ischium,* and *pubis.* The hip, however, describes the projecting part of the body formed by the *acetabulum,* the top part of the femur, and the flesh covering these parts. The acetabulum is a hemispherical articular socket that is formed by the junction of the ilium, pubis, and ischium (see Fig. 3-18, p. 53). Therefore, the hips are really the sides of the pelvis, or haunches. When a person undergoes a hip replacement, the parts involved are the acetabulum (hip socket) and the top of the femur, not the pelvic bones around the waist.

In equine pelvis adjusting, we are mostly concerned with treating the sacroiliac joint, which is where the sacrum articulates with the ilium. It is also possible and helpful to adjust the hip joint by using the long part of the femur as a lever. But for now, here are three methods to adjust the sacroiliac joint by using pelvic contact points.

Method 1: Summit Contact

The name of this method sounds more like a peace agreement between the United Nations and a cold remedy manufacturer, than a chiropractic adjustment. The goal of this method is to release the sacroiliac fixation by contacting one of the *tuber sacrales* (PSIS's). This move is employed if your horse suffers from rear leg lameness, back pain, stifle (true knee) pain, or any other symptom associated with a subluxated sacrum.

Step 1. Static palpation: While standing on a platform, feel the two tuber sacrales as outlined in Chapter 3 (see Fig. 3-22, p. 60). The higher side is your point of contact.

Step 2. Motion palpation: Push down on each tuber and test which one has more spring to it. A springy feeling is a good thing. It means the joint has motion. The joint with less spring is the side of the SI fixation.

Step 3. Muscle palpation: Review muscle palpation for the sacrum as described in Chapter 13. Basically, the side of the pelvis exhibiting tight and tender muscle fibers is the subluxated side.

Step 4. Setup: Stand on a bale of hay on the side opposite the high tuber sacrale. Have your assistant extend the ipsilateral leg (the leg on the same side as the high PSIS, hence, the leg opposite of where you're standing) as far back as possible. Next, place the heel of your hand (pisiform) on the contact (the high tuber) and support your contact hand with your other hand (Figs. 14-1a–b). Stand as close to your horse as possible to maximize your body leverage. Note from the diagram that you'll be leaning over your horse with the top of your breast bone perpendicular to the contact point. Then, apply downward pressure (towards the ground) as well as medial to lateral (middle to outer) pressure.

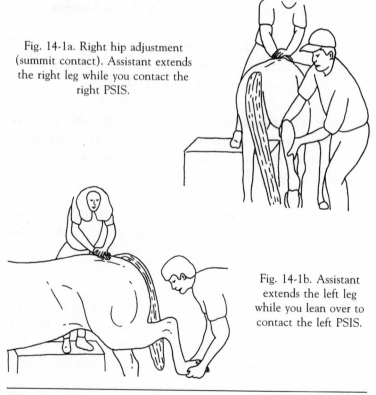

Fig. 14-1a. Right hip adjustment (summit contact). Assistant extends the right leg while you contact the right PSIS.

Fig. 14-1b. Assistant extends the left leg while you lean over to contact the left PSIS.

Step 5. Thrust: With your setup in place, the hind leg extended, and your elbows slightly bent, deliver a sudden and sharp thrust in the direction described in Step 4. Release and recheck your palpation findings. Note: If the horse is acting up and your assistant is unable to extend the leg backward, at least have your assistant lift up the leg a bit to help release the pressure on the SI joint.

METHOD 2: TUBER COXAE CONTACT

You don't need an assistant for this method. The idea here is to use the tuber coxae (ASIS; see Fig. 14-2) as a lever as a mechanical advantage to adjust the fixed SI joint.

Step 1. Static palpation: Same as Method 1.
Step 2. Motion palpation: Same as Method 1.
Step 3. Muscle palpation: Same as Method 1.

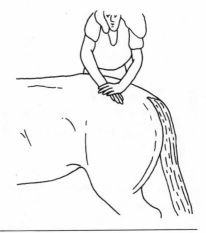

Fig. 14-2. Pushing down the left tuber coxae. The practitioner stands on a platform (bales of hay) on the opposite side and hovers over the horse to reach the contact.

Step 4. Setup: Stand on a platform on the side of the high (subluxated) tuber sacrale (PSIS). Place the heel of your hand on the tuber coxae and support your contact hand with your other hand. Again, the top of your breast bone should be perpendicular to your contact. Next, push (without thrusting) down towards the ground.

Step 5. Thrust: Once your setup is in place, deliver a sudden thrust straight down. This isn't the easiest bone to move. You're going to have to use some body drop as you're thrusting with your hands and arms (your chest drops down concurrently with your arms, adding momentum to the adjusting force). Recheck your palpation findings.

Method 3: Tuber Coxae Contact II

It is possible for the SI joint to subluxate on the *low* side of the pelvis. If this applies to your horse, use Method 3.

Step 1. Static palpation: Palpate the tuber sacrales as in Method 1. Review Chapter 4 for tuber coxae palpation.

Step 2. Motion palpation: Use the same motion palpation procedures here as described in Method 1. The only difference is that the high tuber sacrale will "spring" more than the low one.

Step 3. Muscle palpation: Feel for tighter muscles surrounding the *low* hip side.

Step 4. Setup: Stand on the ground next to the low hip. Place the heel of your contact hand (supported by your other hand) on the aspect of the ASIS that juts out the most, and face towards the opposite (high) tuber sacrale while assuming a sturdy fencer's stance (Figs. 14-3a–b). Have your assistant stand (also assuming the fencer's stance) on the side opposite of you,

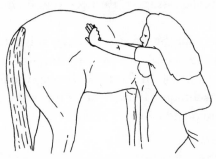

Fig. 14-3a. Tuber coxae contact II. While standing on the ground next to your horse, contact the tuber coxae as shown. Note: Assume a fencer's stance, which braces you during the thrust.

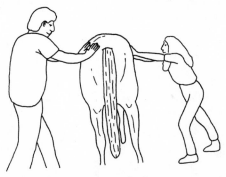

Fig. 14-3b. For the tuber coxae II method, your assistant stabilizes the horse on the opposite side and moves toward the rump—you'll be diagonal to each other.

and have him contact the rump area. You'll be facing somewhat diagonally to each other. Your assistant's job is to stabilize the horse while you're thrusting. Next, apply pressure towards your assistant.

Step 5. Thrust: Once your setup is in place, deliver a sudden thrust towards your assistant. Recheck your findings.

Method 3 is one of the safest and easiest pelvic techniques to apply because it doesn't involve standing on a platform or raising the horse's leg. In the next chapter, you'll learn other easy to apply techniques (how to adjust the tail) which complement the sacrum and pelvic methods.

Chapter 15

Tail Methods

I'm amazed at how often equine chiropractors neglect to check the tail. The horse uses his tail to express emotion, swat flies, and express pain. It is the barometer of the spine. One of the hallmarks of low-back pain, or general body distress, is a tail held tightly to the body. An important part of any equine chiropractic examination is to lift up the tail and appraise its pliancy. A stiff or "fiberglass" tail that feels like it's in the third stage of rigor mortis is one that needs to be adjusted! I like to think of a good tail adjustment as "pulling the rip cord" on the body which releases the rump and back muscles and allows the chute (skeleton) to open and become free. Then again, sometimes I get carried away when I write.

Method 1: Tail Pull

This method is used as a general stress release for the spine. It is a traction technique designed to help low-back and rear leg pain.

Step 1. Static palpation: Check the tail bones (coccygeal vertebrae) for misalignments. They will feel like uneven bony knobs.

Step 2. Motion palpation: Lift the tail up. If the tail lifts up easily and doesn't bend to one side, proceed with the next step.

Step 3. Muscle palpation: Hold the tail with both hands and squeeze it near the base. If the horse reacts by tightening up his rump muscles, that means his tail muscles are in spasm.

Step 4. Setup: Stand directly behind your horse, and grasp the end of his tail with both hands (above the loose hair, on the last few bones).

Step 5. Thrust: With your setup in place, lean backwards, using your body weight to traction the tail. Hold this pose for a few seconds (about 10), then pull sharply towards yourself (Fig. 15-1). Release.

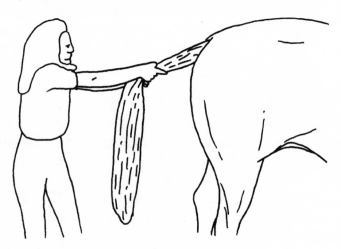

Fig. 15-1. The Tail Pull method.

METHOD 2: TAIL ROTATION

This is also a traction move which helps free up the sacro-coccygeal junction.

Step 1. Static palpation: Same as Method 1.

Step 2. Motion palpation: Stand directly behind your horse, grasp the tail with one hand, and support the horse at the rump with your other hand (Fig. 15-2a). Rotate the tail as if you're "winding up" your horse—first clockwise, then counterclockwise. Ask yourself which direction put up more resistance and make a mental note of it.

Step 3. Muscle palpation: Same as Method 1.

Step 4. Setup: Essentially the same as Step 2. If you found it more difficult rotating the tail clockwise, then stand behind your horse's left rump.

Step 5. Thrust: Position yourself as in Step 4 (on the left rump side). Next, grasp the center of the tail and lift it up as high as you can. Then, in a semi-exaggerated fashion, rotate the tail in a clockwise direction while pulling at the same time (Figs. 15-2b–c). Make about five rotations. **Note:** Don't allow the tail to become knotted up. After each rotation, place the tail down and begin again. Then recheck your palpation findings.

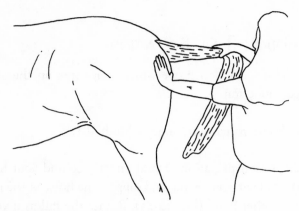

Fig. 15-2a. Tail rotation. This is a combination of rotation and traction. Start by pulling the tail straight back, then clockwaise and then counterclockwise to determine which side puts up more resistance.

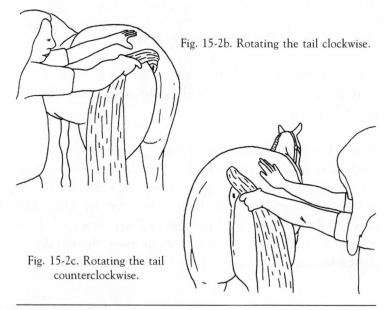

Fig. 15-2b. Rotating the tail clockwise.

Fig. 15-2c. Rotating the tail counterclockwise.

Method 3: Tail Twist

I really don't consider this to be a chiropractic adjustment. It's more of a vigorous, squeezing massage to bring a fiberglass tail back to life. Tail CPR!

Step 1. Static palpation: Same as Method 1. But check for unusual stiffness.

Step 2. Motion palpation: Lift up the tail. If it fights you more than the tightest pickle jar lid, you'll need to use Method 3.

Step 3. Muscle palpation: Feel for extraordinarily tense muscles.

Step 4. Setup: Stand behind your horse on any side, and firmly grasp the base of the tail with both hands (Fig. 15-3). Eventually you will be squeezing all the way down the tail.

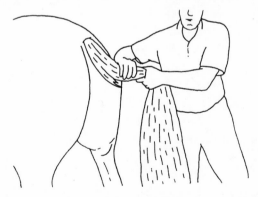

Fig. 15-3. Tail twist move: Grasp the tail with both hands. Twist and squeeze until the joints and muscles become supple.

Step 5. Thrust: There is really no thrust given at all. Once you have the tail firmly grasped with both hands, knead, twist, and squeeze each section until the entire tail becomes supple. Relax every thirty seconds so as to not fatigue yourself. This is hard work. A very stiff tail will take about 5 minutes to soften up. But once accomplished, you will notice a dramatic difference in your horse's demeanor.

Note: Following this procedure I often give the tail some traction (see Method 1) to get the rest of the kinks out. You normally will hear some popping during the first tug.

CHAPTER 16

ADJUSTING THE EXTREMITIES

During my early days at the Palmer College of Chiropractic (in the late 1970s), I used to hear my fellow classmates brag about the terrific spinal adjusting courses taught at the school. One instructor was great with cervical technique, another with thoracic technique, and so on. Only if you listened closely would you hear someone talk about extremity adjusting—how to mobilize the limbs. "What was the problem?" I thought. Why did extremity adjusting take a back seat at Palmer?

The only answer I can provide that makes any sense is that old habits die hard. Palmer was the first, and is therefore the oldest, chiropractic school in the world—the Fountainhead, as it is affectionately known. The success of chiropractic therapy was based on removing pressure off the spinal nerves, not arms or legs. Extremity adjusting wasn't so much taboo as merely second class. It was something a chiropractor would do only if he proved to be an incompetent spinal adjuster. Hogwash, I say! The well educated chiropractor knows the importance of adjusting limbs—not just to make the arms and legs feel better, but to complement the spinal adjustment. Incidentally, it is my understanding that Palmer now embraces extremity adjusting.

Jaw (TMJ) Methods

I had to flip a coin to decide whether the jaw should be included in this chapter or be a continuation of the vertebral methods, which are methods to adjust the *axial skeleton*. The axial skeleton is defined as the skeleton of the head and trunk—including the vertebrae, pelvis, ribs, *and* jaw. In addition, if the jaw (TMJ) is misaligned, the atlas wing on that same side is usually misaligned as well and needs to be adjusted. In contrast, the *appendicular skeleton* includes all the skeletal parts not found in the axial skeleton—arms, legs, and everything attaching thereto. But I will begin this chapter with the jaw nonetheless.

Jaw Method 1

Step 1. Static palpation: The first thing you do is stand directly in front of your relaxed horse (his mouth closed) and look at his bottom jaw (mandible). Since the mandible contains the only freely moveable joint in the head (the TMJ), any noticeable misalignment or deviation from the center would be caused by a lower jaw problem. A misaligned jaw is often caused by improper dental care. Horses grind their food while eating and sometimes develop sharp enamel points on their teeth which must be filed down with a special instrument called a *dental float*. If the teeth are normal, place your hands on each side of the TMJ and note if one side feels bumpier. If so, that means the top part of the mandible (the *coronoid* and/or *condylar process*) is protruding, signalling a deviated mandible (chin/mentum) on that side.

Step 2. Motion palpation: The TMJ moves primarily in a hinge-like fashion with some gliding movement. Reproduce these actions by grasping his mandible at the *interalveolar space* (the section of the mandible void of teeth; see Chapter 3), while stabilizing the opposite *maxilla* (upper jaw) with your free hand. Then, rock the jaw from left to right as well as up and down (Fig. 16-1). If the jaw is deviated to the left, for example, influence the jaw from left to right. If you notice resistance here, the TMJ most likely is subluxated on the left.

Step 3. Muscle palpation: Feel for any tight muscles surround the *temporal* the of the TMJ deviation.

Step 4. Setup: Stand next to your horse on the side opposite the lateral (deviated) mandible. Both of you should be facing in the same direction. For a left TMJ misalignment, grasp the jaw at the interalveolar space with your right hand (this is your

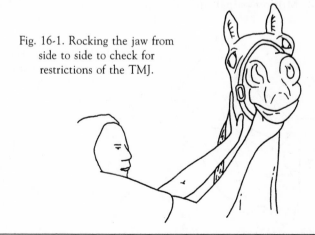

Fig. 16-1. Rocking the jaw from side to side to check for restrictions of the TMJ.

contact hand), and stabilize the top jaw (maxilla) with your left hand.

Step 5. Thrust: With your contact and stabilization hands in place, abruptly, but gently, pull the lower jaw towards yourself (Fig. 16-2). Thrust with your contact hand only. You will usually hear the jaw click into place during this procedure, but this sound can easily be mistaken for the teeth clanking together. **Very important:** More times than not, you will be able to palpate an atlas subluxation on the same side as the misaligned TMJ. If so, adjust the atlas first.

Jaw Method 2

This method is principally the same as Method 1. The only difference is that you will need an assistant.

Step 1. Static palpation: Same as Method 1.
Step 2. Motion palpation: Same as Method 1.

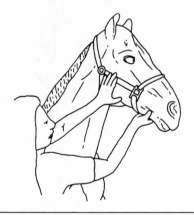

Fig. 16-2. Pulling the jaw towards yourself, away from the restriction.

Step 3. Muscle palpation: Same as Method 1.

Step 4. Setup: Stand on the side of the misalignment and contact the bony area of the mandible just below the TMJ, and support your contact hand with your other hand (Fig. 16-3). Have your assistant stand on the opposite side while stabilizing the occiput (base of the skull) and the upper jaw (maxilla— Fig. 16-4).

Step 5. Thrust: With your setup secure, abruptly thrust lateral to medial (towards your assistant). Again, check your palpation findings and the atlas.

SHOULDER METHODS

Adjusting the shoulder means two things: palpating and treating upper thoracic subluxations, and palpating and treating

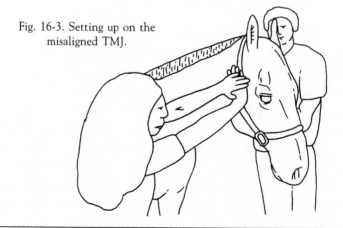

Fig. 16-3. Setting up on the misaligned TMJ.

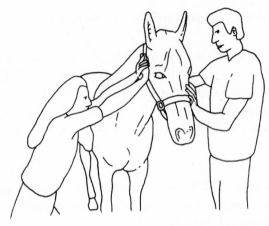

Fig. 16-4. The assistant stabilizes the head and neck on the opposite side while you deliver the thrust on the misaligned TMJ.

scapular subluxations. Before I adjust the thoracics, I will adjust the scapulas. By doing this, I can release considerable mid-back and shoulder muscle tension, which makes upper thoracic adjusting much easier.

Shoulder Method 1 (Lateral Move)

If your horse is weak or sore in one of his forelegs, and it's not due to any diagnosed lameness, then check the affected shoulder. Even though the scapula is not part of the spinal column, I consider a scapular misalignment a true subluxation because it can create many conditions consistent with vertebral subluxations. A misaligned scapula can trap important nerves between the shoulder muscles, such as the *subscapular* and *suprascapular* nerves, which are a vital part of normal ambulation. Since the scapulas are not part of a true shoulder joint (i.e., there's no clavicle, or collarbone), you'll simply be adjusting the scapulas in relation to their surrounding muscles.

Step 1. Static palpation: Locate the scapula as described in Chapter 4. Feel the top cartilaginous border of each scapula, and compare their heights in relation to the upper thoracic vertebrae.

Step 2. Motion palpation: Lift up each foreleg by first bending the knee (carpus). Determine which leg came off the ground easier. The sore leg will put up *less* resistance. Next, check for aberrant scapular movement by placing both hands on the scapula (the upper and lower borders) and have your assistant raise that foreleg (Fig. 16-5). Feel the movement of the scapula and compare to the opposite side. If one side moves less, that will be the side you adjust.

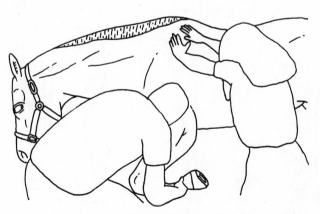

Fig. 16-5. Checking for aberrant scapular motion while your assistant raises the foreleg.

Step 3. Muscle palpation: Feel for tight muscles on the lower part of the subluxated (lateral) scapula. One of the reasons why the scapula is lower on one side is that the tight muscles on the lower part (above the humerus) are pulling it down.

Step 4. Setup: While standing next to the subluxated scapula, lift the affected foreleg by flexing the joints. **Note:** Never try to force the foreleg up. You need enlist your horse's cooperation to do this. "Ask" your horse to lift his foreleg by pinching the insertion of the flexor branch of the *suspensory ligament* above the fetlock (Fig. 16-6a). Once the fetlock joint is flexed, bend the knee by raising the cannon, then grasping the radius with both hands to lift the leg up the rest of the way (Fig. 16-6b). Be

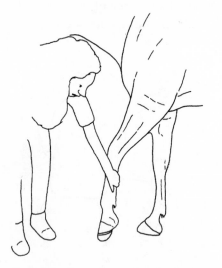

Fig. 16-6a. Preparing to flex the foreleg for the lateral scapular move.

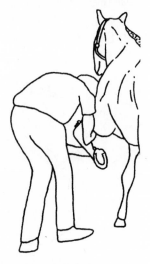

Fig. 16-6b. Lifting up the foreleg.

careful not to contact (squeeze) the knee while performing this move, especially during the thrust. Once the foreleg is fully raised (up to tension), then replace one of your contact hands with your elbow, and hook your arm under the horse's radius (Fig. 16-7). This provides for a much more secure hold on the forearm and positions your body closer to your horse, which saves your own back from distress. Most chiropractors would tell you that the most efficient method of lifting heavy objects is to bend your knees to lower yourself to the object (as opposed to bending forward with your back), then hold the object as close as possible to your chest—the center of gravity. You should never carry heavy objects with outstretched arms. The same principle applies for this adjustment.

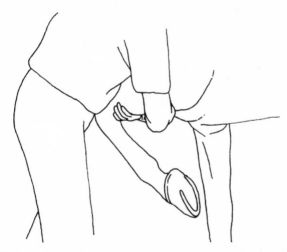

Fig. 16-7. Lateral scapular move. Once the foreleg is flexed, support the leg (below the true elbow) with your elbow and support above the horse's knee with your hand.

Step 5. Thrust: Once your setup is in place, slightly bend your own knees, lift up on the radius until all the joint slack is gone, then thrust up sharply by launching yourself up with your knees, lifting up the radius with your elbow and other hand. Recheck your findings.

Shoulder Method 2 (Medial Move)

This is just the opposite of the lateral shoulder method. In the medial move, one of the scapulas feels higher than the other, and you adjust it by pushing it down. *Medial* implies that the top border of one of the scapulas can be felt closer to the spine or midline than its counterpart.

Step 1. Static palpation: Feel the top borders of each scapula and determine if one of them feels higher relative to the upper thoracics.

Step 2. Motion palpation: Same as Method 1.

Step 3. Muscle palpation: Feel for hard and painful muscles over the high scapula.

Step 4. Setup: Stand on an elevated surface on the opposite side of the high (medial) scapula. As you're hovering over your horse, contact the top border of the "shelf" of high scapula with the heel of your hand (pisiform) and support your contact hand with your other hand (Fig. 16-8). Next, have your assistant raise the affected foreleg all the way up to tension.

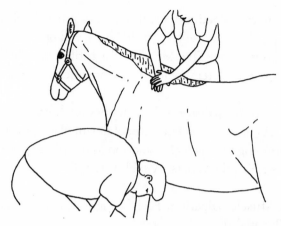

Fig. 16-8. Medial scapular move. Stand hovering over the horse while your assistant raises the foreleg of the affected shoulder.

Step 5. Thrust: With your setup complete, deliver a sudden thrust down towards the ground. Check your palpation findings.

RIB METHOD

There are a myriad of reasons why a horse experiences labored breathing. A fairly common reason is rib pain. During the course of a race, for example, a horse rapidly expands and contracts his rib cage to meet his increased oxygen demands. During this time, one or more of the ribs can become slightly disarticulated from its vertebral attachment. Also, riders who kick the sides of their horse contribute to this problem. Keep in mind that aside from the vertebrae, the ribs also attach to the chest via the sternum.

Step 1. Static palpation: Feel if there is a protruding rib(s) on either side of your horse (Fig. 16-9). A rib will protrude relative to other ribs. Note: The side of the high rib is usually the side opposite spinous laterality for the communicating thoracic.

Step 2. Motion palpation: Trot with your horse for about a minute. As he starts walking to cool down, place your hand on the protruding rib and feel its motion as the ribs expand. Compare this rib to the others. A subluxated rib will expand less.

Step 3. Muscle palpation: Feel for tight muscles surrounding the subluxated rib.

Step 4. Setup: Stand on an elevated surface if necessary. Contact the high rib with one hand (as close as possible to the spine) and support your contact hand with your other hand.

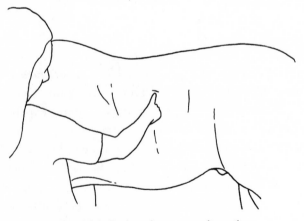

Fig. 16-9. Feeling for a protruding rib.

Then push, without thrusting down towards the ground and slightly towards the tail (Fig. 16-10).

Step 5. Thrust: With your setup in place, swiftly, but not forcefully, thrust in the directions in the previous step. Note: If you feel a high rib next to the breast bone, you can try to contact it and push it up. However, for safety reasons, it is best to simply massage the tight muscles surrounding the high sternal rib.

Elbow Method

To increase restricted joint motion of the elbow, place your forearm in the *cubital fossa* (the space between the end of the humerus and the top of the ulna), and flex your horse's forearm over yours (Figs. 16-11a–b). Hold this flexed position for about ten seconds. This will traction the elbow joint. Do not thrust.

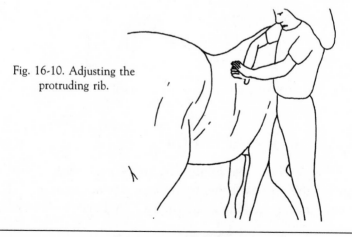

Fig. 16-10. Adjusting the protruding rib.

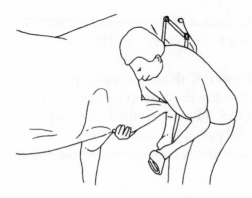

Fig. 16-11a. Testing elbow motion.

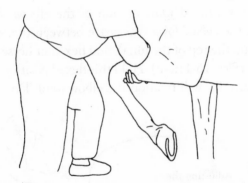

Fig. 16-11b. Placing your forearm in the cubital fossa (elbow joint) to adjust the elbow.

CARPAL (KNEE) METHOD

Freeing up the carpal joints prior to a competition or race is one of the greatest benefits you can provide. I consider this simple move the "unfair advantage." A horse with flexible knees can outmaneuver his competition with less fatigue. "As the knee goes, so go the upper leg muscles." All you have to do for this easy traction move is to bend the knee around your forearm and hold for about 20 seconds (Fig. 16-12).

FETLOCK METHOD

To further increase your horse's front leg mobility, free up the ankle. To do this, simply flex the leg (the knee, too) and grasp the *first phalanx* with one hand, the bottom of the cannon with your other hand (Fig. 16-13a). Hold the cannon still while you pull down (to traction) the first phalange, and open and close the joint (Fig. 16-13b).

Another easy way to mobilize the fetlock joint is to contact one of the two sesamoid bones (see Fig. 3-2) with your thumb and push it down while your other hand tractions and bends

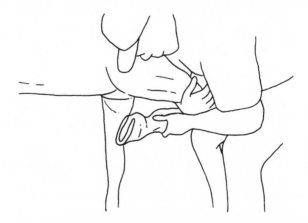

Fig. 16-12. Bending and tractioning the knee (carpus).

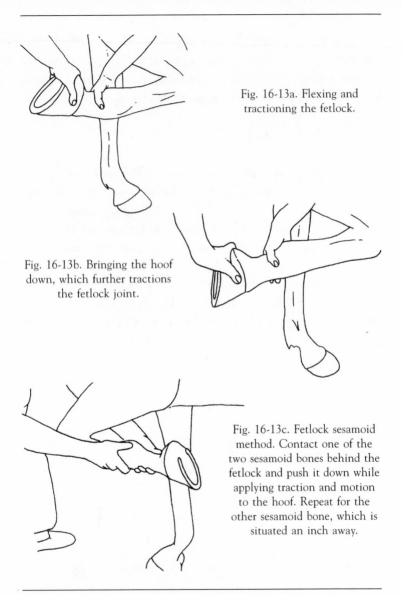

Fig. 16-13a. Flexing and tractioning the fetlock.

Fig. 16-13b. Bringing the hoof down, which further tractions the fetlock joint.

Fig. 16-13c. Fetlock sesamoid method. Contact one of the two sesamoid bones behind the fetlock and push it down while applying traction and motion to the hoof. Repeat for the other sesamoid bone, which is situated an inch away.

the joint by grasping the hoof (Fig. 16-13c). After rocking the joint four or five times, you should feel sesamoid ligaments give under your thumb. That signals the end of the adjustment. (It is also a good time to invoke the traditional magic words, "Open sesamoid!")

Note to the reader: The equine chiropractic methods presented in this book are not an exhaustive account of all currently practiced techniques. However, most of the methods are safe to perform and will provide your horse with much-needed musculoskeletal relief in the absence of professional care.

CHAPTER 17

WHAT ABOUT
INTERNAL DISORDERS?

It's somewhat ironic that the chapter on how to help your horse's insides appears near the end of this book. Most chiropractors seem preoccupied with treating back and neck pain and all but forget about internal conditions. Why? Are they afraid the AMA will raise a condescending eyebrow at them?

The question of why is strictly about money and nothing else. For over thirty years, human chiropractic services have been covered by many major health insurance carriers as well as auto and worker's compensation insurance. Almost all of the diagnostic codes used on the various insurance forms reflect musculoskeletal conditions, mostly lower back and neck pain. There's nothing wrong with this, because chiropractors are in fact back pain specialists. But this just scratches the surface. Chiropractors have adapted to their market to please the patient and please the insurance companies who would otherwise not cover their services if they claimed to help liver disorders.

Chiropractic has clinically been proven helpful for many internal conditions in both people and animals. Among the most common internal conditions helped through chiropractic care are bladder and bowel dysfunction, gastrointestinal disorders, colic in infants, fevers (by boosting the body's resistance), migraines, kidney problems, liver conditions, and asthma, just to name a few. But before you bring yourself or your horse to a chiropractor to have any of the above treated, get a medical opinion first. Chiropractors don't specifically treat these conditions; they find and remove vertebral subluxations that hinder the body's own natural healing powers. Once the subluxation is treated, the body has a better chance to heal itself. But if an internal (visceral) condition is in the acute or crisis stage, then it's too late for chiropractic care, and emergency medical intervention is needed.

These statements represent a general opinion, mainly my own, on the efficacy of chiropractic. But a book of this nature has to side with caution. I don't want anyone to come away from this book thinking that the methods contained in this book can take the place of timely veterinary care. They can't. On the other hand, it's no coincidence that horses and other animals experience miraculous results for many internal problems with a properly delivered chiropractic adjustment.

From the diagrams of the nervous system, notice that specific vertebral areas control or influence certain organs. The lower lumbar region, for example, exerts control over the urinary system. So for urinary and bladder disorders, you would first examine the lower lumbars even though it's quite possible that an upper cervical subluxation could be a factor here.

Where to "Push" for What Condition

While this heading borders on being a little too simplistic, certain ailments do "belong" to definite vertebral segments, or at least predictable areas based on experience, and can be helped through chiropractic care to those areas.

1. Heart Strain: You no doubt have heard the expression "workhorse." A horse works hard and may get fatigued, which puts a strain on its heart. The heart is regulated by several parts of the nervous system including sympathetic and parasympathetic branches of the autonomic nervous system. In general, to provide more nerve energy to the heart, adjust or massage the upper part of the neck (beneath the skull), and the upper and mid-thoracic musculature (1st thru 6th thoracic vertebrae).

2. Lung/Breathing Disorders: I don't have to tell racehorse owners about the importance of lung capacity. But the lungs are just one component of the respiratory system. Other parts include the *nose/nostrils*, which are supplied by nerves originating in the head (cranial nerves) and can, in part, be influenced with upper cervical adjustments; the *nasal cavity*, which is also supplied by cranial nerves; the *larynx* (a structure containing the vocal cords), which has cranial nerve and upper cervical innervation; the *trachea* (breathing tube), with both cranial and spinal nerve (lower cervical and upper thoracic) innervation; and the *diaphragm* (a muscular, membranous or ligamentous wall separating the thoracic cavity from the abdominal cavity), supplied by the *phrenic nerves* which stem from the 5th, 6th and 7th cervical vertebrae. The lungs, partly supplied by the *pulmonary nerves*, will exhibit spinal stress at the base of the skull but mainly the upper and mid-thoracics (T1 thru T8).

2. Constipation and Diarrhea: It is necessary to have your horse checked by a vet for other causes of gastrointestinal disorders, such as parasites, diet, and infections. The spinal areas commonly associated with constipation and diarrhea are the 6th, 7th, and 8th thoracic vertebrae.

3. Ear and Eye Infections: These problems are often seen in small animals, but a horse can be afflicted as well. Cranial nerves control the eyes and the ears; these nerves exit the head near the base of the skull. Therefore, the vertebra most involved in ear and eye infections is the atlas or first cervical vertebra. For chronic infections, you should treat the atlas subluxation weekly for about three months. Of course, your horse should *also* be receiving proper veterinary care for any infection.

OTHER DISORDERS (NOT INTERNAL)

1. Unilateral Nerve Paralysis: While not exactly an internal condition, nerve paralysis is important to note here. An example of this would be sciatica, a rear leg disorder that can cause lameness. The spinal areas involved here are the 4th, 5th, and 6th lumbars as well as the sacrum.

2. Knee (Stifle) Disorders: Subluxations of the 4th and 5th lumbar area often create muscular imbalances that affect the knee. If no patellar (kneecap) injury, bone, or soft tissue disorders are found, then adjust those areas of the lower spine to help the knee.

3. Foreleg Lameness: There are lots of reasons for foreleg lameness in horses. Providing your horse isn't suffering from a commonly seen foreleg condition (i.e., navicular diseases), then look for subluxations at the 5th, 6th, and 7th cervical region as well as the 1st thoracic.

SYMPATHETICS AND PARASYMPATHETICS

The sympathetic and parasympathetic nervous systems each play a part in controlling the internal organs (Fig. 17-1; see also Fig. 3-39). These terms refer to the parts of the autonomic nervous system, which works without your having to think about it (i.e., enabling you to breathe, or digest food while you sleep). The sympathetics are also known as the "fight or flight" nervous system. During times of intense stress, your body releases more adrenalin, giving you supernatural strength despite other ailments such as your arthritic knees, and increasing your heart rate and respiration. This gives you more ability to deal with the situation—to either run or fight. The parasympathetics do just the opposite when stimulated: they calm you down. This is why you shouldn't exert yourself (e.g., swimming) immediately after a meal. Your parasympathetics are busy during digestion, and exercise will kick-start the sympathetics, disrupting the digestive process.

Adjusting the stomach areas found on the parasympathetic chart will stimulate the stomach's function by increasing the amount of acid it produces, while relaxing the muscles around the rectum. The heart will calm down when you adjust the parasympathetic areas and speed up when you adjust the sym-

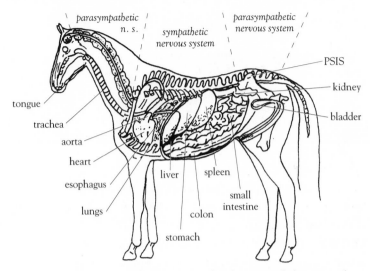

Fig. 17-1. Autonomic nervous system distribution and the internal organs. Study Fig. 3-39 for a better view of nerve locations.

pathetic areas. Therefore, by studying these charts, you'll have an idea of what the effect will be on your horse after the adjustment.

THE METHODS

All of the methods you've learned in previous chapters can be applied when helping internal/visceral conditions. But for those who don't feel confident enough to perform the manipulative procedures, you can still stimulate the vertebrae and reduce spinal nerve irritation by "thumping" the spinal areas (spinouses) with the pinky side of your fist, or vigorously massaging the affected spinal muscles near the vertebra.

CHAPTER 18

WHY DOES A HORSE NEED TO BE ADJUSTED?

There are two notable reasons why I think horses need chiropractic care. The first reason is that when adjusting is indicated, it is a more humane way to treat an animal than drug therapy. Headache pain, for example, is usually extinguished with aspirin, but rekindles when the effects of the drug wear off. People who have been taking aspirin for years often develop stomach and intestinal disorders. To quell their stomach disorders they must take antacids or alter their diets. But why? Why not treat the *cause* of their headaches instead of just masking the symptoms? Chiropractors have known for over a century that most types of headaches successfully respond to chiropractic care, especially an upper cervical adjustment. Once discovered, a person would much rather be under chiropractic care for headaches than constantly poisoning themselves with drugs, suffering from perpetual malaise.

The second reason I think horses should be adjusted is that they get well much quicker than with most other therapies. This, of course, is also more humane. It's true that muscle relaxers calm all the muscles at once—even those that don't need relaxing. This is precisely the point. When a horse suffers from low-back pain the lumbar and hip muscles are involved, as well as a few compensatory areas, such as tight mid-back and neck muscles, which help splint the joints. An equine chiropractor will proceed to adjust the major subluxations then work out the compensatory areas. After all that, the horse still needs muscle tone to *hold* the adjustments in place. A horse under the influence of muscle relaxers is robbed of the necessary muscle tone which should have remained to support the joints. This is why drugs and chiropractic don't mix. The only time I'll ask the vet to administer a relaxant is when the horse is too rambunctious to treat, posing a danger to himself and the chiropractor, namely me!

The methods contained in this book do not take the place of veterinary care. However, for certain musculoskeletal and a few internal conditions, chiropractic is preferred when known to be more effective. For a review of the conditions that favorably respond to chiropractic, see Appendix A.

How do you know which methods to use?

I am happy to report that this is an easy question to answer. Use those methods that best free the fixed joints. And use the methods you feel most comfortable administering. You will learn several techniques for each spinal area. Some require a higher degree of skill than others.

How often does my horse need adjusting?

A horse needs to be adjusted whenever a subluxation is present. Race horses are trained athletes and need to be adjusted weekly. Horses that are ridden frequently should be checked for subluxations after each outing, because the weight of the rider accentuates the stress points of the saddle, namely the front and back of the saddle. "Where the saddle stops, the pain begins."

If during the course of your chiropractic examination you don't notice any fixed joints or spastic muscles, then maybe your horse doesn't need to be adjusted. But at least you checked.

At what point should I consult a vet?

It's best to have a vet examine your horse before you begin administering chiropractic methods, to make sure your horse gets proper treatment for any medical conditions that are past being helped by chiropractic. After that, it's a matter of common sense: check with your vet anytime you feel you're out of your comfort zone in treating your horse yourself.

If I insist on chiropractic care for my horse, but my vet doesn't believe in chiropractic, what should I do?

Get another vet.

Which methods are the most effective?

Believe it or not, I have an answer for this question. But first let me state that with skilled hands, most chiropractic techniques are effective. It just so happens that there are over a hundred styles of chiropractic adjusting—some a little more esoteric than others. To get to the answer, I think the *toggle recoil* and the *ligament push* do the most within the shortest time (see Chapters 10 and 13 for full explanations). I know equine chiropractors who use nothing except these two methods and get amazing results.

How fast can I expect my horse to get better?

It all depends what condition he has and his constitutional vitality. In general, a horse that has the ability to favorably respond to chiropractic care will do so within a few days or weeks. You must consider the limitations of your horse's system. It is possible that your horse may never respond due to destroyed or damaged tissue, in which case multiple adjustments won't help. There are times when you're simply, well, beating a dead horse.

Do adjustments only treat subluxations?

No. To perform an adjustment, the chiropractor's hand contacts a bony part (usually of the spine) and delivers an impulse or thrust with the idea of restoring movement at the spinal nerve exit, namely the intervertebral foramen (IVF). Aside from giving the body shape and structure, the bones are mostly sites for muscle attachments. Therefore, by putting the whole bone in motion, you are essentially moving all or most of these muscle attachments, which frees up a broad range of joints, including the IVF. This is why a chiropractor can have you "loose" in minutes, while a massage therapist can take up to an hour. I know there are many other benefits of massage therapy. But I think you get the point.

Are there any animals who don't benefit from chiropractic care?

Yes: Dead ones. The rest can *all* benefit from chiropractic care, to varying degrees. Animals with medical conditions, however, should also be receiving competent medical care (see the next question).

If my horse is lame due to a hoof disease, should he be adjusted?

This is the best question of all. To the astonishment of some vets, I have treated many horses suffering from laminitis (a.k.a. founder), which is defined as an inflammation or edema of the sensitive *laminae* (fibers which attach the coffin bone to the hoof wall). Note that I said, "I have treated many horses suffering from laminitis"—I didn't state that I treated the laminitis itself. There's a big difference. Horses who are lame due to hoof diseases fall out of alignment all the time. Why not keep them comfortable while they're healing? I also treat human patients who have cancer, but I don't treat the cancer. Removing subluxations strengthens the body's overall healing capabilities. A very sick person or animal needs every advantage. So while I'm not treating the horse's laminitis, I *am* treating the horse who's suffering from laminitis.

Can an adjustment hurt my horse?

Any time you make physical contact with a patient, whether human or animal, there is always an element of risk. An osseous adjustment is accomplished by applying a sudden force to a joint. If you push too hard where you shouldn't, yes, you can hurt your horse. But it's unlikely you'll injure your horse if you use only your hands to adjust, and not mallets, two-by-fours, or other medieval devices.

Should my horse feel better immediately following an adjustment?

Usually not after the first adjustment. In fact, your horse's muscles may be a bit sore after the initial treatment. The muscles take time to get used to their new position, and the horse will show some sensitivity. Once your horse is accustomed to being adjusted, he'll be less sore and for shorter periods.

Should I adjust all of the subluxations I find?

The answer is yes, but perhaps not all during the same session. What I like to do is concentrate on the major subluxations, which are associated with the primary complaint, then let the horse rest for a few hours. If the horse is too sore, I'll do some light muscle or stress point work, and again let him rest a while. Here's where you have to use your better judgment. If the horse is getting tired of *you*, it's time to quit for the day.

How will I know if my horse is relaxed?

It's a funny little phenomenon, but a horse will lick his lips following a satisfying adjustment. Not only have I witnessed this thousands of times, but every equine chiropractor I know reports the same observation. Some equine massage therapists see this as a toxin release.

Chiropractic methods are the major focus of this book, but I've also included a chapter on equine muscle therapy, mainly the stress points associated with muscle injuries. Much of this information is derived from *Beating Muscle Injuries for Horses* (Hamilton Horse Associates, 1985), by Jack Meagher (pronounced "Mar"), one of the country's leading sports therapists.

THREE CASE HISTORIES

1. Many years ago, I adjusted one of the best-natured Thoroughbreds this world had to offer. Rusty Jet was a five-year-old gelding with the heart and soul of a lamb but the speed of a cheetah. Funny thing about Rusty—he was a good earner but he never won a race! That's right. He never finished first, but he placed more than any horse I can remember. Rusty would start the race fast, and stay fast until the final eighth of a mile. Sometimes he would be a full three lengths in front of his nearest rival. But the second he sensed another horse was gaining, he would slow down and

let that other horse win. Most people who saw Rusty race said he felt sorry for the other horses.

During the late summer of 1989, Rusty started to slow a bit and was finishing third and fourth—still in the money, but not up to his potential. When I trotted him, I noticed his left hip appeared to be slightly higher than his right, and his right front foot would violently stomp on the ground for no apparent reason. His trainer did not report any injuries, and the vet examined him and said he was fine—maybe just a little overworked. I examined his entire spine and found two major subluxations: his left sacroiliac and right scapula. Upon further interrogation of the trainer, I learned that Rusty had been transported out of state a few weeks before and had endured a very long and bumpy ride. That explained everything. He was trying to balance himself in the trailer for several hours, and his muscle cramped. So the first thing I did was massage those areas and worked out a few stress points around his hip and shoulders. I then administered a lateral scapular move on his right shoulder, tractioned out the right carpus, and then I adjusted his left sacroiliac joint using a summit or PSIS contact. After four adjustments over a two-week period, Rusty was as good as ever— finishing second like his old self!

2. About four years ago, a human patient of mine asked me to look at her 7-year-old mare, Katie, who had recently started a habit of rearing up and throwing her off while riding. I drove over to her barn and watched Katie walk and trot. She looked fine. I then palpated her neck, with-

ers, and lower back. When I pressed my fingers into the sixteenth thoracic, Katie let out a loud whine and reared up—I mean almost vertical!

The diagnosis was easy. Part of the saddle was digging into that area of the back. I asked my patient about the saddle. She told me she had just bought it and that it cost about a thousand dollars. Price, however, doesn't have much to do with the way a saddle fits. I adjusted the subluxated vertebra and applied the Ligament Push (Logan Basic Technique) during each of four visits over a three-week period. After the third week, Katie was no longer tender, and her owner was able to ride her again. And of course, a new saddle was bought for Katie from a reliable dealer. That did the trick.

3. Moe was a 21-year-old retired Standardbred who seemed to be wasting away. His caretaker said he hadn't been eating much for a few weeks and the vet was contemplating his demise. Horses this old generally get arthritis, become slow, and appear depressed because no one pays much attention to them.

I palpated Moe's neck, shoulders and back and felt the usual drooping signs of aging muscles. The most notable finding was tenderness over the right jaw (temporomandibular joint, or TMJ). Also, when I touched his right atlas, he whined and tried to head-butt me. When a horse does this, he's in pain. I found out Moe had been ridden about two months earlier by a robust right-handed man who was a little rough. This bit of information was important, because a horse's head and neck tend to hurt on the side of the rider's dominant hand. After the examination, I adjusted the right TMJ and the atlas on the right using the toggle recoil move. Moe immediately showed signs of relief by drinking water and grabbing a mouthful of hay. But there were other problems which I couldn't fix. Since his TMJ and atlas had been subluxated for a long time, his teeth were wearing asymmetrically and needed to be floated— which they were, and Moe completely recovered.

Horses can develop sharp enamel points caused by grinding their teeth while eating, or by an atlas subluxation creating irregular muscle pulling on an imbalanced jaw. If a horse's jaw is misaligned due to an atlas subluxation, the problem may not be noticed for months, if ever. That's why it's important to check your horse on a regular basis for vertebral subluxations to help prevent these problems before they fester into a crisis.

HAZARDS ON THE ROAD

The past few years of my life have been spent on the road working the seminar circuit. I used to conduct these seminars with Dr. Bill Inman, a Seattle veterinarian who is both a very intelligent chap and a little on the serious side, like Jack Webb of Dragnet, "Just the facts, ma'am." Dr. Inman and I would meet at various cities around the country and teach animal chiropractic methods to other professionals. The seminars were well advertised and we usually had several dozen prepaid registrants. These events usually come off without a hitch. But once in a while....

The Unexpected Pregnancy

At just about every seminar, we invite the doctors to bring in some of their own pets or their clients' pets to demonstrate the chiropractic techniques. Last year in Manhattan, we must have had a dozen dogs and cats scampering around the meeting room during the seminar. One of the attending vets asked a client to bring in her dog, a 3-year-old male Italian Greyhound, who was suffering from a rather undignified bladder condition and wasn't responding to medication.

"Joey" was a cute, well-muscled little black dog who couldn't have weighed more than 8 pounds—at least 7 of which was macho. I imagined an earring hanging off his left ear and a half-opened flea collar. "Yo, Adrienne!"

Dr. Inman examined and then adjusted Joey with the spring-loaded device. Then I had a crack at him. Instead of using an osseous move (joint manipulation, complete with sound), I used the Logan Basic move (pushing the ligament underneath the tail, above the anus). Joey wasn't too happy about this, but after a couple of minutes, the adjustment was over and he swiftly ran to the other side of the room and hid under a table.

The rest of the seminar progressed as planned, and we left for home Sunday evening. About six weeks later, I received a frantic phone call at my office.

"Hello," I said, wondering who was yelling at me.

"This is Joan Mills," the voice on the other end screeched.

"Who?"

"Joan Mills."

"Am I supposed to know who you are?" I asked.

"You should," her breathless voice said. "You adjusted my dog Joey at the seminar."

"I did?"

"Yes. You and that other fellow. Inman, I believe."

"Where?" I inquired. "We adjust so many dogs."

"In New York," she countered. "Remember Joey, the little Italian Greyhound with the bladder problem?"

"Oh, yeah. Now I remember. So how's he doing?"

"Not so hot," Joan said.

"Is his bladder still out of sorts?" I asked.

"No," Joan said. "His bladder is working fine and he hasn't had an accident in weeks."

"So what's the matter?"

"Toni's pregnant," she said with a little hysteria in her voice.

"Who's that?"

"Joey's sister," Joan said. "She's gonna have a litter."

"Mazel tov," I said in a forced Yiddish accent. "But I thought those relationships only happened in the South."

"No, wait," Joan begged. "We thought Joey was sterile and couldn't make puppies, so we didn't foresee any problem leaving Toni with him."

"So what do you want me to do about it?" I aked suspiciously.

"Well," Joan continued, "I thought maybe that adjustment you gave Joey could have activated something. You know. His sperm count. Is that possible?"

"Well, it's not impossible," I said. "The bladder and the reproductive organs have various functions in common. So, sure, it's possible."

"Then you're responsible for the pups," Joan said.

"What are you talking about?" I snapped back. "Are you implying that I'm the father of those puppies?"

"Don't be ridiculous," Joan countered. "I'm just saying that you didn't tell me the adjustment could stimulate sperm production."

At this point I thought someone was playing a joke on me. Not that I don't deserve it. Heaven knows I do my share of kidding. But this lady sounded as frantic as a skydiver with a broken parachute a hundred feet from the ground.

"I don't know what to tell you," I continued. "But don't forget, Dr. Inman adjusted Joey, too." Not that I was selling out Dr. Inman, but if by some miracle she could prove paternity, I'd only have to pay half the puppy support until the kids turned two and a half (that's eighteen in people years).

"Yes," she sarcastically chortled, "you both may very well be responsible."

"That could be," I said. "But if the whelps are born with a little goatee [like Dr. Inman's], I insist they be raised Catholic."

"Dr. Kamen," Joan said. "I don't think you realize how important this is to me. The breeder sold us these dogs because we promised not to breed them ourselves. He too was convinced that Joey couldn't reproduce. And now this. What am I supposed to do about it?"

"Furthermore," I said, continuing from my last statement, "I will not pay for an out-of-state college."

Apparently, that was the end of the conversation. I heard nothing but silence on the line and figured that was that. But that wasn't the end. An hour later, Dr. Inman called me, saying he had just heard from this same nut.

"What did you tell her, Bill?"

"I told her to pull Toni out of school and move out of town to save her reputation. Then she hung up on me."

"What do you think she'll do," I asked.

"What else can she do?" Bill said during an uncharacteristic jocular moment. "Hold Toni's paw and count the contractions between deliveries."

Only in New York!

Denver International Airport

There's one thing I've noticed about traveling—people in public places would rather not be surprised.

In the spring of '96, Dr. Inman and I were conducting a large seminar in Denver. Our seminars are held on Saturdays and Sundays, so we usually fly into town the Friday evening before to prepare for the weekend event. Since I'm from the Chicago area and Bill is from the Pacific Northwest, our flight schedules would rarely coincide and it was unusual for us to meet at the airport. But Denver was different.

The minute my plane landed in Denver, I and the rest of the gazelles headed for the baggage claim area to collect our precious freight before some imaginary local derelict got to it first. (Incidently, to assure no one steals your luggage all you have to do is paste a sticker on your bag that says, "Property of the Department of Infectious Diseases.") Anyway, as I politely bulldozed through the herd towards the conveyer belt, I saw Dr. Inman struggling with the bulky footlocker which contained a beat-up dog skeleton—his prized demonstration tool.

"Bill," I said, surprising him with my presence.

"Dan. When did you get here?" Bill inquired.

"Ten minutes ago. I see you're still lugging Old Yorick around."

"Yea," Bill said. "It's easier than you carrying around a horse."

Actually, I do carry around a horse, but it's a small plastic model that snugly fits into a medium size traveling case.

"You know, Bill," I said as we were dragging our stuff towards the hotel shuttles. "You should really consider adjusting horses by hand."

Dr. Inman is primarily known for adjusting small animals with the little spring-loaded adjusting device commonly known as an activator.

"Naw," said Bill. "Too physical."

As we neared the shuttle, I told Bill I had to go to bathroom since I had had a lot of coffee on the plane and wouldn't last the ride to the hotel.

"So do I," Bill said, as we started walking to the toilet.

I kept on talking, thinking Bill was walking with me as I entered the lavatory. I was nonchalantly describing how to adjust a horse's neck by hand while I was busy at the urinal.

"You see, Bill. It's really quite simple," I loudly said while speaking to the white concrete wall in front of me. "You grab the beast by its long, sturdy neck, and stretch it until you let out all the slack, then give it a firm twist until you feel a snap. Just be careful it doesn't bite you. These creatures are ticklish sometimes and very head-shy. But I really like it. This method is the most efficient way of getting the joint to move. Sometimes I do it thirty times in a day. Did you ever try this, Bill? Bill?!"

My peripheral vision failed me this time. It wasn't Bill who was standing next to me. It was some elderly, bearded gentleman who resembled a disgruntled looking Jack Kevorkian. I stopped mid-stream and quickly aborted my equine adjusting instructions. Dr. Death peered over the urinal partition, and looked down at my hands to see what I was talking about.

I zipped up post haste and sheepishly walked over to the sink to wash my hands. While I was drying my hands under the hot-air blower, I noticed "Jack" staring and shaking his head with a "you meet all kinds of weirdos" look on his face. As I was leaving the facility, he nudged up against me and said, "Can you teach me to do that?" We both chuckled a little and walked out the door.

I saw Bill talking on the phone. I waited there until he was finished.

"I thought you had to go to the bathroom too."

"I did," said Bill. "But I remembered I had to call Wendy (his fiancé) first."

I told Bill about my experience.

"Let this be a lesson to you, Dan." Bill said. "That wouldn't have happened if you just treated small animals."

Maywood

I know what you're thinking. Where, for the love of Mike, is Maywood? I'll tell you. Maywood is a city near Chicago. It is also the name of a harness racetrack located there. This anecdote, incidently, doesn't really qualify as an "On The Road" story, but it concerns horses and my brush with the underworld.

About eight years ago, an acquaintance of mine, Harry Shelton, owned two very capable harness horses and stabled them at Maywood Park. Harry was a well-connected guy with a reasonable amount of money. About 47 years old at the time, Harry had all the outside appearances of a normal suburban man who liked to have a good time. He was a fun-loving sort with a wife, an ample paunch (him, not his wife), two almost-grown daughters, a modern house, and a Jaguar. His thick, horn-rimmed glasses and frizzy black hair completed that eastern, Gene Shalit look. But there was a problem. You see, Harry didn't seem to have a job. He had money, but no job. How did he get it?

Harry loved to play the big shot, and as long as he doled out the cash, everyone would coddle him. Once or twice a month during the evening racing season, he would pick me up at my office and chauffeur me to Maywood Park, then sloppily park his car two feet from a valet, hand him the keys and a ten spot, then quickly flash his pass (not that it was necessary) at the man guarding the entrance. As we briskly walked towards the sky boxes, the air would be dotted with several, "Hi Harrys" until we were escorted to our seats. Harry would flash a big wad and have a waiter bring him his drinks and run his bets for him.

Harry won big and lost big. He got good tips and won with those, but lost betting on his own selections. At the end of the evening he picked up all the tabs, worked the room for a few more minutes, then left with the same celebrity status as when he arrived. So, exactly how *did* he make his money?

During the ride home from one of these excursions, I noticed he made one phone call after another. I didn't know the people he called, but it was easy to deduce they were his "customers." Things like "the Bears and five," could be heard throughout his conversations. In other words, Harry was a bookie. On a good day, he kept over thirty thousand in cash in his car and would sometimes make his payoff drops on the way home. But though I knew he was into this bookie thing, I didn't know how much until his house of cards collapsed one day.

"Doc," he asked me, "I need a favor."

The haunting lilt in his voice when he asked me to do him this favor signaled trouble.

"What, Harry," was my pensive reply. Whatever it was, I didn't want to end up sleeping with the fishes.

"I got myself in a little too deep at the Park, and I need to get my horses out of the stalls."

"What do you mean?" I asked in disbelief. "How much do you owe them?"

"About ten G's. And I haven't got it now."

"What happened to all of your cash?"

"Gone," said Harry. "Dolphins wiped me out last week."

This wasn't good. But there was more to the story. Not only was Harry in debt booking, but he owed some drug money, too. Had I known he was involved in drugs at the time, I would have dropped him like a bad habit.

"What do you want me to do, Harry?"

"Doc, it's really easy," he assured me. "All you have to do is walk into the barn and lead Mountain Man and Wendall out of the grounds."

"Why can't you do it yourself?" I anxiously retorted.

"Because they know who I am. The front girl was told not to let me in. Doc, you've got to do this for me."

"Is that all you need? Just your horses?"

"No, the tack, too."

"The tack?" I shot back. "How much do you have back there?"

"Whatever there is," Harry said. "Just load it all on Mountain Man."

"I don't know about this, Harry. Sounds a little risky."

Did you ever have that "I'm going to the gallows" feeling? Well, I did. And I didn't like it. There was something very unholy about this situation. But I agreed to do it the next day and we made the necessary arrangements. The plan was that Harry would borrow a trailer that would accommodate two horses, and hurry them off to his friend's barn in Woodstock, Illinois, about 60 miles away-as the crow flies! The deal was that I simply had to walk the horses over to this trailer and leave, stat! But that's not what happened.

About eight o'clock the night of the heist, I casually walked over to the barn where Mountain Man and Wendall were stabled. Absolutely no one noticed or paid any attention to me. I acted like I owned the joint. I opened Wendall's stall, led him out, then Mountain Man's stall and ushered him out as well. I piled all of Harry's tack and anything else I suspected was his on Mountain Man's back, just as planned. With a lead in each hand, I sauntered out of the barn, and through the gate I went. Again, completely unnoticed. "Piece of cake," I thought to myself. "This puts me right up there with Billy The Kid!" And there in the distance, I saw Harry waving his arms at me as he stood by the trailer which was hooked up to his Jaguar.

"Doc, over here," Harry shouted.

I walked the geldings over to Harry, took a deep breath, and handed him the reins.

"Here you are, Harry. They're all yours."

"Wait, Doc. We've got a problem," Harry said in an apprehensive whisper. "I could only manage a one horse trailer."

"So," I said. "What's that got to do with me?"

"Well," Harry continued, "I need you to baby-sit one while I haul the other one to Woodstock."

"You're kidding," I yelled in disbelief. "Where?"

"Here," said Harry. "You're gonna have to hold one here for a couple of hours until I get back."

"No!" I protested. "Absolutely not. And it's not going to be just a couple of hours. We're talking at least three."

"Doc, you have to. I've got nobody else. Just do it."

My heart sank to my feet. I had gone along so far with his plan and felt obligated to see it to the end. But I had an eerie feeling I was going to take the fall for this. So there I was. It was already dark and I was standing outside in the cold with an unpredictable horse five feet from a busy city street. I watched as Harry started his car and made his way out of the grounds. I looked at Wendall, my obligation, and counted the minutes until I was free—whenever that would be.

It's hard to explain, but there's something very spiritual about standing with a horse next to a city street. Sort of frontier-like. The only thing I missed was not seeing *Miss Kitty* at the saloon. But my bubble soon faded when the minutes turned into hours. It was 10:45 at night and the last race had just finished. As the remaining diehard fans filed into their cars and drove away, I was still standing there with Wendall. By 11:15 the area was deserted, except for an occasional car that would slowly pass while its driver gawked to see the lunatic standing there with a horse for no apparent reason. But I wasn't scared, yet. You've heard of a watch dog. Well, I had a watch horse! The tough looking guys who passed by just kept going. However, it was getting late, and Wendall was getting tired and hungry.

At about midnight, I had a brief encounter with three "gang" looking teenagers. These thugs came complete with neck tattoos, nose piercing, weird hair sculptures, and cocky attitudes. As these rowdies were approaching, I was thinking about Redd Foxx, "This is the big one, Elizabeth." The leader of the pack walked right up to me. I knew he had to be the leader since he had fewer teeth than the other two and he was eager to show off in front of his army.

"Hey, man," the leader said in his best Sweat-Hog brogue, "what'cha got there?"

"Here?" I nervously replied. "This is Wendall. I was asked to keep him here for a few minutes until the Department of Animal Sanitation (whatever that is) arrives. This poor fellow has J.E.A., Juvenile Equine AIDS, and has already infected two other horses and three grooms."

At that precise moment, Wendall had a severe "restless" attack. He was ornery from not eating and let loose a loud whine and reared up about three feet in the air.

"Get down," I shouted hysterically. "He's about to strike!!"

You should have seen those punks run. I think the leader of the pack produced some new graffiti near his wallet.

After that bit of excitement was over, I kept Wendall busy by pacing him back and forth along the curb. To give myself a break, I periodically tied the leads to a stop sign and stretched my legs. I had nothing for him to eat and he was getting restless. It's funny, but at least five squad cars passed by and none of them stopped to ask me what I was doing. I suppose it's perfectly natural to see a guy standing with a horse next to the street at 2:00 in the morning. Yes, 2 a.m.!

Finally, at 2:13 a.m., Harry's Jaguar engine pierced the night's silence and I saw the wobbly trailer lumbering towards me.

"Where the hell have you been?" I screamed.

"Relax, Doc. Mountain Man gave me a hard time when I got there. Jerry (his trainer in Woodstock) wasn't there and I had to handle him myself. You know me—I'm no horseman."

"Oh, for Pete sake, Harry. I'm cold and miserable. Let's get Wendall in there and I'm out of here."

Harry drove off with Wendall and I finally got to go home. I didn't get much sleep that night because I had to get up at 8:00 to see my 9:00 appointments. When I arrived at my office at 8:45, my receptionist, Janis, was already there and so were two new faces.

"Howdy," I said to the two strangers who were sitting in my waiting room. I hurriedly scooted past them and headed for my private office. Janis stepped in and told me about the men.

"Dr. Kamen," Janis said, "those two guys want to talk to you about a horse."

"Who are they?" I asked.

"I'm not sure," Janis said. "But they mentioned something about a missing horse. They want to talk to you."

"Good grief," I told Janis, "Someone must have spotted me at the track last night. Did Harry call?"

"No," Janis said. "The phone hasn't rung all morning."

I fixed my tie and walked back to the waiting room.

"Yes, gentleman. What can I do for you."

They introduced themselves as Len and Chuck, and said they were the owners of Mountain Man and Wendall.

"What?" I said in shock. "Harry Shelton owns them. But what's that got to do with me?"

"Tom Horton (another horse owner whom I did some work for) saw you standing out on First Street last night with two horses. This morning we noticed our horses were gone and we suspect you took them."

"I didn't exactly take them," I said. "I was helping Harry transfer them to another barn."

"But they weren't his to transfer," Len said. "If we don't get them back today, we're going have you and Harry arrested."

"But I didn't know you owned them. Harry said they were his."

"Harry is a liar and a crook. He owes me and Len five thousand for past gambling debts and the track another ten for boarding and medical bills. He signed off on those horses last week."

I didn't know what to do. I was thinking that Harry probably had made arrangements to sell the horses and I was left holding the bag.

"I'll tell you what," I said, "I'll call Harry and you can talk to him yourself." They agreed.

I tried to call Harry, but he was no where to be found.

"Guys," I said. "I'll try calling him in an hour."

"No good," said Chuck. "We need to get the horses now."

I thought about this situation for a minute. These guys weren't going to have me arrested. They were involved in gambling themselves and who knows what else. I'm sure they didn't want the police involved. My only way out of this was to tell them where the horses were and to fight it out with Harry. My whole livelihood was at stake here. Worse yet, I could get dead!

"Look fellas," I said, "Why don't you get the horses yourself. I think I know where they are."

They agreed to take a look, but only if I went with them. The last thing I wanted to do was drive in the same car as these goons. I talked my way out of going with them, citing that I had to see patients the rest of the day. They begrudgingly agreed to drive out to the barn themselves, but said they'd "get back to me."

The rest of the day was a blur. My head was in a fog and I found it difficult to concentrate on rendering quality care. Seven o'clock rolled around and I was just about to leave for home when the phone rang.

"Dr. Kamen?" I answered.

"Doc," shouted the voice at the other end. "My horses are gone."

It was Harry. Apparently Chuck and Len had successfully retrieved their property.

"Harry," I interrupted, "slow down."

"Doc, did a couple of guys visit you this morning?"

"Yea, Harry. They did."

"What did you tell them?"

"Harry, Tom Horton saw me with the horses last night and told these two guys where to find me. They said Mountain Man and Wendall belonged to them. Is that true?"

"Oh, Doc. You shouldn't have told them where they were. Yes, it's true, but I needed the money. I'm in big trouble now."

"Wait a minute," I angrily said. "You had me wait five hours last night in the cold to help you *steal* those guys' horses?"

"You don't understand, Doc."

Immediately after, Harry said, "Doc!" I heard some commotion over the phone and then. . . silence. I tried calling back, but the line was busy. I went home and worried the whole night. I'm not a drinking man, but I took a couple of shots of Crown Royal, which was left over from a New Year's party two years before. I went to work the next day and tried calling Harry again. I called him at home, at the stable, and I even tried calling a few friends of his. Nothing. That night after work, I sat in front of the TV eating a light snack, when all the sudden my jaw dropped a foot.

"Oh, my, my, my," I screamed to my wife. "Sharon, turn on Channel 5. You'll never guess who just got arrested!"

Yep, it was Harry. There he was on TV, with a full frontal view of him being hauled into the police station. But not for horse thieving. He was arrested for attempted murder! I found out later one of his drug deals went sour and he tried to pay a guy three thousand dollars to bump someone off.

The shock and excitement wore off after a few weeks, Harry's lawyer made a deal with the D.A., and Harry was sent to prison for fifteen years. It was all over the papers. About a month after that, I got a call from Chuck.

"Is this Dr. Kamen?"

"Yes. To whom do I have the pleasure?" I said in an upbeat voice.

"This is Chuck. Remember? Me an Len visited your office a couple of months ago to get our horses."

"Yea, I remember," I said with a little tremble in my voice.

"Well, Mountain Man is running again, but according to his trainer, he's been having back pain. I understand you can help him. How's about meeting us for dinner tomorrow night as my guest at the clubhouse?"

I was visibly startled by the invitation and then composed myself.

"I'd love to," I said. "But I have to wash my hair tomorrow night. Maybe some other time."

Appendix A

Chiropractic Care for Equine Conditions

The following conditions affecting horses can, in part, be treated with chiropractic care. But **without exception,** horses suffering from the disorders listed below should be under veterinary care since many of these maladies can be career-ending or life-threatening.

Navicular Disease (Distal Sesamoid)

- Primarily a disease of the forefoot, and a common cause of forelimb lameness affecting the flexor surface of the bone.
- Quarter Horse and Thoroughbreds, especially geldings, appear to be most at risk. Rare in ponies and Arabians.
- Causes include heredity/breeding (small feet compared to body size), prolonged working on hard surfaces, or improper trimming of the feet (causes increased pressure of the deep digital flexor tendon across the navicular bone which increases the forces across the bone). Also cited as possible causes are ischemic necrosis (tissue death due to decreased blood supply), and arterial thrombosis (blood clotting).
- One or both feet may be affected. Usually worse the day after hard work.
- Other characteristics of navicular disease include short peri-

ods of remission after rest, "walking on eggshells" (landing on their toes to avoid heel strike), stumbling, and signs of shoulder lameness (shortened stride).

- The treatment for milder cases includes rest, corrective shoeing, anti-inflammatory medication or a palmar digital nerve block. In severe cases, a neurectomy (cutting the nerve leading to the heel) is performed to control pain. The prognosis is guarded in all cases. The chiropractic approach is meant to supplement the medical treatment by relieving back pain. Since a shortened stride and a stumbling gait are signs (due to pain), regular scapular adjustments should be made to relieve shoulder stress, as well as upper thoracic adjustments. Light to moderate traction (by hand) of the foot may be applied if the inflammation is not too severe. Also, light to moderate traction of the carpus may be applied. All surrounding trigger points should be worked out (with a light touch) along the leg and shoulder. The brachiocephalic muscle is a common site for trigger points. These procedures should be performed no more than twice a week and only if the horse is allowed to rest.

Roachback and Swayback

- Though these conditions are uncommon, they are more common in the foal and are considered to be defects of the spine, i.e., congenital scoliosis.
- Improvement may be spontaneous and complete.
- Problems with the gait are usually NOT seen.
- One reason why roachback (exaggerated kyphotic curve or hump) is not observed in mature animals is because foals

afflicted with this are often destroyed, since their usefulness is perceived as limited (riding, working).

- Swayback, when congenital, is due to hypoplasia (incomplete development) of the intervertebral articular processes (the flat surfaces where two vertebrae meet to form a joint).
- These two conditions are sometimes seen in adult horses and will cause weakness of the back muscles.
- Swayback (lordosis, or hollowing of the back) is observed at the vertebral levels T5 through T10; Roachback (kyphosis/hump) is observed between L1 through L3 vertebral levels.
- In sheep and goats, swayback, a.k.a. enzootic ataxia, is a neurological disease (lesions of the spinal cord and brain stem/myelin deficiency), and is noticed in the early stages of life (birth to 4 months) exhibiting signs of hindlimb ataxia (loss of coordination), paresis (partial paralysis of the limbs) and sometimes tetraparesis (total paralysis of the limbs). This condition is associated with copper deficiency in the dam and offspring and may be successfully treated with copper sulfate.
- The chiropractic approach does NOT include adjusting the affected areas of the spine for roachback or swayback. Your goal is not to return the curvatures to normal, but rather to make the animal more comfortable. Myofascial techniques (pressure points and trigger points) are appropriate here as is Logan Basic/Ligament Push.

Sweeney

- Definition: Atrophy of two muscles located over the scapula, the supraspinatus (which extends the shoulder joint) and the infraspinatus (which abducts the arm and rotates it laterally); usually caused by damage to the nerve supply to these muscles (suprascapular nerve for both muscles). This nerve arises from the cranial section of the brachial plexus (C6, C7, and C8). The rest of the brachial plexus includes nerves arising from T1 and T2. Sometimes the pectoral nerve is involved with no pectoral muscle atrophy. The pectoral nerve arises from C7 and C8 spinal nerves.

- An abnormal gait is generally not seen early on—until severe muscular atrophy. The abnormality noticed first is difficulty with shoulder extension.
- Cause may be an injury to the suprascapular nerve (direct blow or fall).
- Dramatic clinical observation is a sharp outline of the scapular spine with chronic cases.
- This condition causes a loose shoulder joint and is often mistaken for a shoulder dislocation. A "slipped shoulder" is observed at the affected leg when the animal takes a semicircular step, and the shoulder joint moves laterally upon weight bearing.
- Medical treatment includes anti-inflammatories, or surgical intervention by notching out the scapula to relieve tension on the nerve. Rest is also indicated.
- Chiropractic therapy is often successful with 4 to 6 months of treatment. Adjusting the lower cervical and upper thoracic subluxations as well as administering the lateral scapular move is indicated. It takes several months of treatment because it takes that long for the damaged nerves to resupply the atrophied muscles.

- Trigger point therapy, massage, and electrical therapy are also beneficial.
- Polo ponies are sometimes affected due to collisions during competition.

Cauda Equina Neuritis

- Severe and progressive lower motor neuron (LMN) disease, primarily affecting adult horses. A lower motor neuron is that part of the peripheral nervous system that connects the central nervous system with the muscle to be innervated.
- Areas affected include the sacral portion of the spinal cord nerves and associated nerve roots.
- Possible involvement of cranial nerves (nerves originating inside the head—specifically nerves V, VII, and VIII), producing signs such as head tilt, nystagmus (rapid and involuntary movement of the eyeball), and facial paralysis.
- Lesions associated with this condition resemble allergic neuritis—suggesting autoimmune polyneuritis (inflammation of several nerves at the same time).
- Clinical signs include: urine scald (dripping urine on the inner thighs due to urinary incontinence), rubbing the perineal area (the area in front of the anus extending to the fourchette of the vulva in the female and to the scrotum in the male), and constipation. Paralysis of the tail, the bladder and anal sphincter are also found. Additional signs may be noted in the male horse, including dropped penis (inability to retract the penis).
- If both sacral nerve signs as well as cranial nerve signs are noticed, then the diagnosis is probably cauda equina neuri-

tis. If just the sacral signs are noted, then check for possible sacral fracture (a veterinary procedure).

- Medical treatment is generally not curative, and the prognosis is dim. Bladder and bowel evacuation are the main concerns.

- Logan Basic is the most effective chiropractic technique for bowel and bladder control. This may help prolong the inevitable. It is best to teach the owner to do this procedure since it has to be performed on a daily basis.

Wobbler Syndrome

- Wobbler syndrome, also known as Cervical Vertebral Malformation or Equine Sensory Ataxia, is seen in the first through second year of life.

- Clinical signs include incoordination (a neurological sign) in young horses, especially Thoroughbreds. They appear clumsy in the hind end, with occasional forelimb spasticity.

- Narrowing (stenosis) of the vertebral canal (C5–C7) and spinal cord compression (demyelination is the main pathological change) contribute to the neurological signs. The involved vertebral area are the mid to lower cervical vertebrae (C4–C6).

- Causes are mixed. Heredity, high protein intake, and injury to the spinal cord at the mid- to lower cervical area are possible causes.

- Medical treatment includes surgery, but is costly and the prognosis is poor.

- Chiropractic treatment should NOT include osseous adjusting to the cervical spine. Adjusting the lower spinal and sacral subluxations won't hurt, but may not improve the condition. Myofascial therapy around the tight cranial muscles, especially at the suboccipital region will temporarily soothe the horse's distress. Logan Basic is also indicated with sometimes impressive, but again, temporary results.

Atlanto-Occipital Malformation

- Found in Arabian Horses (both sexes). Hereditary condition.
- Noticed at birth, this defect compromises the spinal cord due to narrowing of the vertebral foramen of the atlas. This results in cranial cervical spinal cord compression.
- No discernible atlanto-occipital joint, as the atlas is fused with the occiput. Causes ventral displacement of axis and a short dens.
- Signs include: inability of the foal to stand, or ataxia if the foal can stand; difficulty nursing, since neck extension is limited while standing; an audible "click" is heard when the head is moved (due to the atlanto-axial luxation); spastic thoracic limbs upon walking; neck appears to be "stiffly extended;" palpably smaller atlas wing.
- Prognosis is guarded to poor. A similar disorder has been described in Holstein cattle.
- This condition cannot be cured. Chiropractic care can be rendered only after suitable X-rays have ruled out a severely narrowed atlas foramen. The atlas should not be osseously adjusted, rather, the lower cervical vertebrae (C3 through C7) should be gently manipulated for the purpose of reduc-

ing neck stiffness. Myofascial techniques are recommended.

Coxitis

- Also known as osteoarthritis of the hip, resulting from inflammation of the coxofemoral joint.
- Causes usually include trauma (falls or lying down in the stall too long on one side); lameness will be noted upon standing and walking.
- In severe cases, the horse will "carry" the leg. In less severe cases, the horse will raise its hindquarter up as weight is applied to the affected leg. Semicircular motion of the leg coupled with a shortened stride is observed. The toe may be worn from dragging. The animal will sometimes stand with the limb partially flexed, the stifle turned out, and the point of the hock turned inward. Muscle atrophy will sometimes occur around the affected limb.
- Even though most types of treatments provide little relief (intra-articular steroids may help some), chiropractic care may be the most beneficial. Trigger point/myofascial therapy around the coxofemoral joint and surrounding muscles usually provides several days of pain relief as does Logan Basic. The PSIS contact to adjust the SI joint is also helpful, and may be applied up to three times per week.

Trochanteric Bursitis ("Whirlbone" Lameness)

- Inflammation of the bursa that lies beneath the tendon of the middle gluteal muscle as it passes over the point of the hip.
- Common in Standardbred racehorses. Causes include fall-

ing on the hip; straining of the tendon during racing or training; direct blow to the hip, such as a kick.

- Horse will show pain upon applying pressure over the greater trochanter. The affected leg is often rested in flexion. The horse will walk on the inside of the hoof wall, which wears down the medial side of the hoof.
- This condition is often confused with hock lameness or hip-joint abnormalities. In chronic cases, the muscles on the side of the affected hip become atrophied, and the croup takes on a flat appearance.
- Medical treatment includes rest, and injecting the bursa with anti-inflammatories/corticosteroids. The chiropractic approach also includes rest, but also myofascial therapy is indicated, as well as a PSIS contact to relieve pressure on the gluteal muscles. Logan Basic should also be applied on the affected side.

Muscle and Ligament Strain

- Soft tissue damage is the primary cause of back pain in horses.
- Typically involves the longissimus dorsi complex of muscles which act to extend (dorsiflex) and laterally flex the spine. Another site often affected is the supraspinous ligament, which runs down the middle of the back and adheres to the thoracic and lumbar spinouses. Because of this ligaments various tendinous insertions relating to the longissimus dorsi complex, it is subject to the same strains as the muscle.
- Among the numerous causes of strains, the most common would be injuries which occur during riding and exercising.

- The major areas of injury/strain include the caudal withers, and cranial lumbar regions. Note: These body areas are the points just in front of and behind the saddle area.
- There are various medical approaches to muscle and ligament strains ranging from rest to surgery. The chiropractic approach is to adjust all of the surrounding subluxations and apply myofascial/trigger point techniques on or around the affected muscles or ligaments—noting the contraindications (tears, wounds, etc.)

Carpitis

- Inflammation of the joint capsule (acute or chronic). Also known as "Sore Knee" or "Popped Knee." Must rule out carpal bone fractures in order to diagnose.
- Acute conditions are more common in Thoroughbreds that train on hard surfaces; also seen in hunters and jumpers. Lameness is due to distention of a joint capsule/swelling.
- Medical treatment includes rest, draining the fluid, corticosteroids, and in severe cases, surgery.
- Chiropractic methods include gentle manipulation of the carpus (flexing the carpus over your arm and applying light traction) and gentle lower cervical manipulation. This should only be done only after a thorough medical diagnosis to rule out the usual contraindications (fractures, exostosis, bleeding, etc.).

Stringhalt

- Also known as "springhalt." Horse exhibits a spasmodic overflexion of one or both hindlimbs. Sometimes this spasm is so severe that the foot touches the belly, then is suddenly slapped down to the ground. Backing the horse out of the stall will exaggerate this sign.

- The etiology of this condition is not readily known, but most of the literature suggests two possible causes: lesions (peripheral neuropathy) of the sciatic, peroneal, and tibial nerves; and lathyrism (sweet pea poisoning).

- Not common in North America. Much more common in New Zealand and Australia, especially during late summer and early autumn.

- This condition often does not inhibit the horse's ability to work. Prognosis is guarded to good.

- If intoxication is the suspected cause, the treatment is simply to remove the horse from his usual stall, isolating him from the legumes.

- Other medical treatment includes surgery (cutting a portion of the lateral digital extensor tendon), large doses of thiamine and phenytoin (a barbiturate-related substance used as an anticonvulsant in the treatment of grand mal epilepsy and in focal seizures).

- Chiropractic treatment includes adjusting the lower lumbars and SI joint and applying Logan Basic, since this would relieve pressure on the sciatic nerve. Look for and treat the trigger points around the buttocks and hamstring areas. This, of course, should be done in conjunction with proper veterinary care.

Sacroiliac Subluxation

- Not to be confused with the chiropractic definition of subluxation. In this case, it means a rupture or tear of the sacroiliac ligaments due to injury which often results in a sacroiliac dislocation and hindlimb lameness.
- Also known as "sacroiliac strain," "sacroiliac arthrosis," and "hunter's bumps." It appears as though the hip on one side has shifted and is trying to poke through the skin.
- Shifting of the hindlimbs and dragging of the toe of one or both hoofs is often noticed, as is a higher sacral tuber (PSIS). Also noted is smaller gluteal muscles, asymmetry of the croup, and an off-centered tail. Pain upon applying pressure medial to the tuber coxae (ASIS) is sometimes noted. Also, the horse will be reluctant to ventroflex the back.
- Common in Standardbreds and jumpers.
- Medical approach usually includes anti-inflammatories, and rest, (usually successful for treating pain after several months).
- Chiropractic treatment is very successful to relieve pain after the ligaments have healed. Osseous sacroiliac adjustments, trigger points and Logan Basic are the methods of choice. Note: The dislocated sacroiliac joint cannot be corrected with chiropractic care.

Femoral Nerve Paralysis

- The femoral nerve supplies the muscles that extend the stifle (knee joint). Paralysis of this nerve prevents the horse from extending this joint. Also seen in cattle following a difficult birth (affects the calf).

- Affected horse is observed in a crouched position. The affected leg is unable to support weight. Also noted is atrophy of the quadriceps femoris, and hypometria (short steps).
- Causes include general anesthesia (forcing the horse to lie on the nerve for long periods during surgery); overextension of the limb during exercise, causing an over-stretching of the femoral nerve; and injury caused by a kick.
- Medical treatment consists of anti-inflammatories and rest, depending on the severity and cause. The prognosis is guarded to poor. Chiropractic care includes adjusting the SI joint, and myofascial/trigger point therapy along the muscles of the affected hindquarters and leg.

Radial Nerve Paralysis

- The radial nerve supplies the extensor muscles of the forelimb, allowing the horse to bear weight on the leg. Paralysis of this nerve impedes these functions.
- The primary cause is trauma (often associated with a fracture of the humerus). Another cause is general anesthesia (if the horse was placed on its side on a hard surface during a lengthy surgical procedure).
- If the nerve is completely severed, there is no cure and the horse must be destroyed.
- A common medical treatment is to use anti-inflammatories.
- Chiropractic care is successful in less severe cases. Trigger point therapy, and adjusting the lower cervical and upper thoracic subluxations should be considered. Light but frequent adjustments to the carpus are also indicated.

Horner's Syndrome

- A partial interruption of the nerve supply to the eyes and head will produce clinical signs known as "Horner's syndrome." (Spinal cord function reflected in the head is sympathetic innervation. With Horner's syndrome, there may be lesions of the intermediate grey column from T1 to T3.)

- The clinical signs in horses include constriction of the pupils and protrusion of the third eyelid (drooping of the upper eyelid is sometimes seen). Sweating on the face and neck of the affected side is also noticed.

- Causes of Horner's syndrome include localized infections, perivascular injection, foreign bodies, and trauma to the neck.

- Chiropractic treatment includes adjusting the atlas (toggle is the preferred method). Contact the side which presents with the most signs (sweating, drooping of the eyelid, etc.). Also, osseously adjust T1 through T3. When successful, results are noticed within a few days.

Appendix B

Notes on the History of Animal Chiropractic

When a janitor named Harvey Lillard stepped into an old and musty office in the midwestern river city of Davenport, Iowa, he walked into history. It was 1895, the year chiropractic was born. Founding father Daniel David (D.D.) Palmer, a Canadian-born magnetic healer, discovered the chiropractic principle by accident after Mr. Lillard complained of hearing loss. Seventeen years earlier, Mr. Lillard told him, he had felt a snap in the back of his neck while lifting something at work, and had been almost stone deaf since then. Detecting a misaligned vertebra in back of Mr. Lillard's neck, D.D. Palmer snapped it into place, and Mr. Lillard's hearing soon improved.

Following this startling discovery, D.D. Palmer wondered whether adjusting the spine might not be the key to curing other ailments. He knew there were direct and indirect spinal-nerve links to all of the body's organs. Therefore, he reasoned, a pinched spinal nerve leading to the stomach might lead to gastrointestinal conditions, and so on with all the other spinal-nerve-to-organ connections.

Apocryphal or not, this story is the chief reason why the

chiropractic profession has been the object of the medical community's incessant ridicule, most of which originally stemmed from irresponsible publicity surrounding this story. Claims of deaf cures were advertised throughout the Midwest. People flocked to Davenport to see the new "miracle healer."

The word "chiropractic"—composite of the Greek *cheir* (hand) and *praktos* (done), hence "done by hand"—was also born in 1895. The Palmer School of Chiropractic was created in the same year, and the profession soon began to flourish. However, it wasn't until D.D.'s son, Bartlett Joshua (B.J.) Palmer, began to practice that chiropractic became a household word, thanks to his charismatic style and business savvy. Unfortunately, his outrageous claims of curing everything short of rigor mortis tarnished the credibility of an incredible discovery.

Early chiropractors were often jailed for practicing medicine without a license. This was clearly an attempt by organized medicine to derail the young profession's momentum. Still, chiropractors thrived. The public wanted an alternative to drugs and surgery. Today, all fifty states license chiropractors, thanks in part to the sophistication and quality of chiropractic educational institutions. It takes at least six years of rigorous training to become a licensed chiropractor. Note: Chiropractic is also practiced worldwide. Most of the chiropractors who practice in other countries were educated here, but several fine chiropractic schools are located in various parts of the world, including Europe, Japan, Australia, and Canada.

Unsurprisingly, the first chiropractor to practice on animals was D.D. Palmer. Along with his son B.J., he organized within the Palmer School of Chiropractic a course in animal adjusting, and even printed a two-color diploma to issue to those who might complete a comprehensive one-month course of study. Although my search of the literature has produced no evidence of anyone actually receiving one of these DCV (Doctor of Chiropractic Veterinary) diplomas, the Palmer College of Chiropractic (previously the Palmer School of Chiropractic) has a copy of this document in their archives. Also uncertain is the year this course was offered, although it is generally accepted that D.D. Palmer adjusted animals and taught his techniques around the turn of the century. (He died in 1913 at age 68.)

Early chiropractors practiced on animals primarily in order to arrive at a proof of the central feature of their new science, the subluxation theory—i.e., that a pinched spinal nerve caused "dis-ease" in the corresponding organ or function. During the beginning years of the profession, B.J. Palmer wanted to demonstrate that the adjustment had more than a placebo effect, as had been charged by the medical community. Unfortunately, the clinical accounts of his successes with animals were largely anecdotal, and B.J.'s work on animals has all but been ignored. To make matters worse, the *Journal of the American Medical Association* stated in its issue of September 17, 1921, "If chiropractors are wise they will confine their malpractice to humans; it is safer." This quip was printed after the AMA learned that Palmer School graduates were working on animals. The article continued, "That men ignorant of the body and its processes should treat the ailments of men, women and children is apparently a small thing; human life is the only thing involved. But that ignoramuses should trifle with the health of a horse or a hog is an outrage; that is property."

Despite the AMA's efforts to discredit the profession and protect the lower life forms, animal studies have often been used to bolster the subluxation theory. When an animal died, the cause of death—such as heart failure, liver, kidney disease, and so on—would be determined. Then a surgical dissection of the spine was made to see if there was any spinal-nerve impingement linked to the animal's condition. And indeed, there often appeared to be a connection between the diseased organ and the corresponding impingement.

Even as the AMA demanded proof of the subluxation theory, it refused to approve any sort of chiropractic activity, including scientific experiments. And while the AMA has never had the legal authority to control the practice of chiropractic, its opinions have always carried enormous political weight, which translates into public opinion. Chiropractors are often asked whether they are now accepted by the AMA, and the answer is always the same: "It doesn't matter." The AMA is a private professional association that sets standards of practice for its members—M.D.s, not D.C.s.

The discovery of chiropractic in 1895 created a new element on the health-care periodic table. The first reaction of Western medicine was to purge this beast from the forest. But as the years passed, the medical community has had to acknowledge that chiropractic is here to stay. Even chiropractors themselves started to believe they were here to stay! The reason? Results. As long as sick people and animals continue to get well, chiropractors will be in demand.

Recently, there has been a proliferation of well-documented

scientific research that deeply investigates all the components that add up to the subluxation theory. The research includes studies in biomechanics (joint and muscle movement), comparing the effects of soft to moderate thrusting (i.e., the "adjustment") and the effect it may have on its target, such as an internal organ or muscle. The analogy has been made to a light switch: by turning on the spinal nerve, you light up the organ. It's up to the chiropractor to find the "switch" in the spine and turn it back on.

There is still relatively little literature available on animal chiropractic, however. This is partly due to the fact that chiropractors, as compared to M.D.s, have always struggled to keep themselves afloat financially, and have therefore had almost no time to work for extra credit. And while veterinarians have always had more than enough to do treating the everyday emergencies that arise in their practices, chiropractors have had more than enough to do just holding onto their licenses to practice. Because most states do not allow chiropractors to work on animals, animal chiropractic remains a closet profession.

One of the early animal chiropractors was Dr. Myles A. Medford, born in 1926 and still going strong. Dr. Medford was discouraged by his experience studying veterinary medicine: he didn't like the huge classrooms or the staff shortages at Coffeyville College in Kansas, and besides, a medical education was expensive. This turned out to be a lucky stroke for animal chiropractic. After attending the Palmer School, Dr. Medford began adjusting animals in 1954 and is recognized as a pioneer in the field, having organized a series of one-on-one workshops with other chiropractors and developed many of the current adjusting techniques. He still maintains a refreshingly youthful enthusiasm regarding the future of animal chiropractic.

In a thought-provoking man-versus-beast comparison, Dr. Medford once stated, "Chiropractic adjustments of the animal kingdom can and do release much more nerve force in quadrupeds than in man. This is due to man allowing his educated intelligence to rule his existence. Educated intelligence in man has all too often overruled the simple rules of innate" ("innate" being synonymous with "life energy"). In other words, Dr. Medford doesn't believe in animal hypochondriacs, whereas people can be talked into—or talk themselves into—believing they're sick. (Every time we learned about a new disease in school, someone in our class would come down with it the next day!) Conversely, animals don't have to believe in chiropractic in order for it to work.

At present, none of the fifty states allows chiropractors to practice autonomously on animals. There is, however, a growing number of veterinarians taking a second look at the benefits of chiropractic for animals. The wave of the times is, after all, natural health care. Given the choice, the informed health-care consumer would rather treat his or her body with pure food, clean water, and exercise than be mistreated with chemicals and the high cost of trying to compensate for an unhealthy lifestyle.

Domesticated animals would surely make the same choice if they could. It is up to us to see that there *is* a choice.

Appendix C

Where to Find Animal Chiropractors

It's actually getting easier to find a professional person in your area who is proficient in animal chiropractic techniques. Through various teaching programs, such as the seminars I conduct, more chiropractors and veterinarians are including animal chiropractic as part of their regular services.

If your veterinarian or chiropractor does not perform this service, or can't due to legal restrictions, then you may call my office at 1-800-742-8433. I have amassed a list of over 500 doctors nationwide who have some expertise in adjusting animals, including horses.

You can also visit my website, www.animalchiropractic.com, to learn more about my current projects and conferences, as well as to find additional information on animal chiropractic, including video clips of adjustments available for download.

For those chiropractors who wish to practice with a vet but don't know which ones would be amicable to this business arrangement, then contact a vet who is a member of one the holistic organizations listed below. They tend to be more sympathetic towards chiropractic.

1. American Holistic Veterinary Medical Association
   2214 Old Emmorton Rd.
   Bel Air, MD 21015
   (410)569-0795

2. International Veterinary Acupuncture Society (IVAS)
   c/o Meredith L. Snader, VMD
   2140 Conestoga Road
   Chester Springs, PA 19425
   (303) 258-3767

3. Toxicology Hotline for Animals
   University of Illinois College of Veterinary Medicine
   2001 S. Lincoln Ave.
   Urbana, IL 61801
   1-800-548-2423

4. California Holistic Veterinary Medical Association
   c/o Beth Wildermann, DVM
   17333 Bear Creek Rd.
   Boulder Creek, CA 95006

5. Dr. Bill Inman, D.V.M.
   7769 58th Ave. NE
   Seattle, WA 98115
   (206) 523-9917

BIBLIOGRAPHY

1. Gatterman, Meridel I. *Chiropractic Management of Spine Related Disorders*. Williams & Wilkins, 1990.

2. Getty, Robert. *The Anatomy of the Domestic Animals: Volume 1*. W.B. Saunders Company, 1975.

3. Kamen, Daniel. *The Well Adjusted Cat*. Brookline Books, 1997.

4. Oliver, John E., & Lorenz, Michael D. *Handbook of Veterinary Neurology*. W.B. Saunders Company, 1993.

5. Stephenson, R.W. *Chiropractic Text Book*. Palmer School of Chiropractic, 1927.

6. *The Merck Veterinary Manual*. Merck & Co., Inc., 1991.

7. Siegal, Mordecai. *UC–Davis Book of Horses*. HarperCollins, 1996.

8. Meagher, Jack. *Beating Muscle Injuries For Horses*. Hamilton Horse Associates, 1985.

9. Hawcroft, Tim. *The Complete Book of Horse Care*. Lansdowne Press, 1983.

10. Stashak, Ted S. *Horseowner's Guide To Lameness*. Williams & Wilkins, 1996.

11. Hourdebaigt, Jean-Pierre. *Equine Massage*. Howell Book House, 1997.

12. Rooney, James R. *The Lame Horse*. Melvin Powers Wilshire Book Company, 1974.

13. De LaHunta, Alexander. *Veterinary Neuroanatomy and Clinical Neurology*. W.B. Saunders Company, 1983.

14. Cleveland, C.S. *Chiropractic Principles And Practice Outline: Volume IV*. Cleveland College of Chiropractic, 1951.

Marketplace

1. **Videos** on animal adjusting (dogs, cats, or horses). These 90-minute VHS videos demonstrate easy-to-do animal chiropractic methods. Anatomy as well as adjusting techniques are covered. $49.00 plus $4.50 s&h. Illinois residents add 8¼% sales tax ($4.05). Specify dog, cat, or horse.

2. **Metal mallet.** $159.00 (lowest price available) plus $4.50 s&h. Illinois residents add 8¼% sales tax ($13.12).

3. *The Well Adjusted Dog.* $16.95. The first book on animal chiropractic; available in most bookstores or from Brookline Books, 1-800-666-2665. Signed copies may be ordered from Dr. Kamen at the address below.

4. *The Well Adjusted Cat.* $13.95. Available in most bookstores or from Brookline Books, 1-800-666-2665. Signed copies may be ordered from Dr. Kamen.

Send check payable to:
Kamen Chiropractic
1121 Highland Grove Dr.
Buffalo Grove, IL 60089
or call 1-800-742-8433
www.animalchiropractic.com

INDEX

ABOUT THE AUTHOR

Dr. Daniel Kamen was born on June 18th, 1956, in Chicago, Illinois. He has been practicing chiropractic since 1981. His father is a highly respected anesthesiologist; his mother, a gifted artist. Dr. Kamen's original animal chiropractic organization, "Animal Crackers," produced animal chiropractic educational materials, which taught others how to adjust dogs and horses.

Dr. Kamen lives with his wife, Sharon, of eighteen years, along with their three sons, Jeffrey, Gary and Kevin. He makes his home in Buffalo Grove, Illinois. Dr. Kamen has been featured on many TV, radio, and newspaper stories concerning his work with animal chiropractic. He currently is on tour, teaching a professional as well as a lay lecture seminar on animal chiropractic (horse and dog adjusting). His hobbies include playing the piano and chess (master level).

~ ~ ~

Visit www.animalchiropractic.com to learn more about Dr. Kamen's current projects and conferences, as well as to find additional information on animal chiropractic, including video clips of adjustments available for download.

ABOUT THE AUTHOR